Acknowledgments

I'm grateful, as usual, to Brad Kearns, who always goes above and beyond the call of duty and gets the job done faster than anyone else. My husband, Paul Spencer, did all the mathematical calculations that my brain couldn't handle, along with invaluable legwork that led me to numerous athletes and a slew of interesting training trivia and athletic records. I also appreciate the help of Sarah Bowen Shea, Richard Motzkin, Liz Neporent, and the twenty-four accomplished athletes who took the time to offer thoughtful responses to my questions.

Expert Contributors

Glenn Gaesser, Ph.D., professor of exercise physiology and director of the kinesiology program at the University of Virginia; coauthor of *The Spark* and author of *Big Fat Lies.*

Liz Neporent, M.A., C.S.C.S., board member of the American Council on Exercise; author of *The Ultimate Body: 10 Perfect Workouts for Women* and *Fitness Walking for Dummies*; coauthor of *The Fat-Free Truth.*

Cynthia Sass, M.A., M.P.H., R.D., spokesperson for the American Dietetic Association; adjunct professor of nutrition at the University of South Florida, Tampa; coauthor of *Your Diet Is Driving Me Crazy.*

The Ultimate
Workout Log

The Ultimate Workout Log

An Exercise Diary for Everyone

THIRD EDITION

SUZANNE SCHLOSBERG

HOUGHTON MIFFLIN COMPANY

Boston New York 2005

To all the exercisers who have kept this log going
for more than a decade!

Contents

Introduction to the Third Edition

You asked for it—you got it!

The log you're holding has undergone a major makeover since the second edition, thanks to all the loyal users who have taken the time to post suggestions online or to e-mail me personally. Redesigning the log wasn't tough, since just about everyone made the same request: add more space. OK—done! The third edition has everything you've asked for—more room for strength-training notes, a designated section for yoga or Pilates, a bigger box for nutrition notes, and a special "Daily Wrap-up" area to record overall feelings and impressions. If you've used previous editions of this log, you'll notice the most significant change right off: there's now an entire page for each day of the week.

But the page design isn't all that's new. The third edition is filled with intriguing nuggets of research and fitness trivia that you can toss around at your next Spinning class or group hike. Any idea how the dumbbell got its name? Or what about the origins of the term "bikini"? You'll find out in Week 5 and Week 8, respectively. And guess who can run faster: a world-class sprinter or a kangaroo? The answer appears in Week 2. Plus every Saturday there's a mini nutrition quiz. (Which has more calcium: a cup of yogurt or a cup of spinach? Find out in Week 4.) You'll cap off each week with words of wisdom from an accomplished athlete.

WHY KEEP A LOG?

This log may look different from previous editions, but its purpose remains the same: to help you stay motivated, achieve your fitness goals, and feel a sense of accomplishment. Whether you're aiming to finish your first triathlon, set a personal bench-press record, or simply fit back into jeans you've outgrown, your log will help you get results. It will reveal patterns in your training and help you discover how much exercise—and how much rest—is right for you. And it will prod you to set goals that are concrete and realistic while devising strategies to reach them.

Can a bunch of blank pages really do all that? "The mere fact of writing something down makes you more committed to it," says sports psychologist Robert Weinberg, Ph.D., a professor at Miami University in Ohio, who has done extensive research on goal setting and athletic performance. When it comes to setting goals, Weinberg's motto is: "Ink it, don't think it!" I second the motion.

Many of the world's best athletes are diehard believers in recording their goals and tracking their workouts. "Keeping a training log is invaluable," says 2004 Olympic marathoner Alan Culpepper. "It is the best way to truly dissect and reflect on those things that worked well and those that did not. It also keeps you honest. You have to have some way to monitor your training to make sure you're not neglecting or overemphasizing one area." As Culpepper points out, it's so easy to forget what you did two weeks ago, or even two days ago.

Of course, you needn't be a world-class athlete to learn from your log. In fact, newbies may even have the most to gain. Jayne Williams, author of *Slow Fat Triathlete*, records not just her mileage but also her sleep quality, fatigue, soreness, stress level, and overall well-being. "It makes me pay attention to what's going on in my life as a whole," Williams told me. "If I've been up half the night watching cheesy movies, I shouldn't be surprised that I don't feel fresh for my run the next day."

Your log not only will help you adjust your training but also will

2

boost your confidence by reminding you of all that you've accomplished. Deena Kastor, a 2004 Olympian and the American record holder in the women's marathon, highlights her exceptional workouts so they'll stand out when she flips back through her log before a competition. "I get energized to bring back the emotion of the great days," she says.

Champion wheelchair racer Jean Driscoll considers her training journals to be nothing less than personal treasures. "They are a record of what I've done, where I've been, who I am, and where I can go," says Driscoll, a two-time Olympic silver medalist and eight-time Boston Marathon winner. "They are as much a training partner to me as my teammates are."

My own log served as a confidence booster not long ago, after I broke my tailbone—ouch!—in a cycling accident. When I learned that I'd be forced off the bike for six weeks—double ouch!—I worried, as injured exercisers usually do, that my hard-earned fitness was going to vanish overnight. I moped and whined for a few days, but then, in a more rational moment, I flipped through my log and saw how consistently I'd been training for many months. Clearly, I'd built a solid base that was likely to carry me through. I reminded myself that you can't lose your fitness the way you can lose your car keys!

Once my tailbone healed, it did take me three or four weeks to get back up to speed. At first, even cycling short hills left me gasping for breath, and there were days when all I wrote in my workout log was "Ugh!" and "#$%*$#!" But before long, I was back in form, making notes like "felt strong!" and "awesome workout!"

My hope is that you'll have plenty of awesome workouts to record in this log. I welcome feedback on this new edition.

Suzanne Schlosberg
suzanne@suzanneschlosberg.com

Setting
Your Goals

Superstar swimmer Megan Quann has a remarkably colorful bedroom door. That's because it's plastered with the 101 lifetime goals she has set for herself, all printed out on colored paper in different colored inks. "I never want to forget my goals," says Quann, a two-time Olympic gold medalist who holds the American record in the 100-meter breaststroke. "I want them always in front of me, ready to be accomplished."

Most of us don't need to take the concept of goal setting quite that far, but there's no doubt you'll achieve more if you step onto the elliptical trainer or the tennis court with a sense of purpose than if you wander aimlessly through your workouts. That's why a significant amount of space in this log is devoted to recording your goals and assessing whether you've reached them. A wealth of research and experience has shown that certain types of goals work better than others, so consider the following tips as you fill out the goal sections in your log.

MAKE YOUR GOALS SPECIFIC AND MEASURABLE

Consider this: In a three-month study conducted at Miami University in Ohio, researchers told a group of exercisers that their goal was to increase by 20 percent the number of abdominal crunches they could do; they simply told a second group, "Do your best." Not surprisingly, the group with the concrete objective performed a significant 10 percent better than their rudderless peers. In other studies, health-club exercisers who set specific workout goals had significantly lower dropout rates — as much as 20 percent lower — simply because they had a specific target.

The same idea applies to nutrition goals, too. In a nine-month Australian study, subjects who were told to eat four servings of fruits and four servings of vegetables daily ended up eating more fruits and veggies than did subjects who were simply instructed to eat more produce.

Even if your ultimate goals are nebulous — maybe you're striving to be more fit, slim down, be healthier, or have more energy — it's important to choose specific objectives for your workouts. For example, you could aim to complete a 100-mile bike ride or run 30 minutes on the treadmill at a 9-minute-per-mile pace or even show up at your yoga class three times a week for a month.

Keep in mind that not all concrete exercise goals involve mileage or a revved-up heart rate. "To keep yourself mentally fresh, set goals that are kind of off-the-wall," suggests Jayne Williams, creator of the hilarious and inspirational Web site www.slowfattriathlete.com. "Set a goal that you'll say hi to a new person at every track workout."

MAKE YOUR GOALS CHALLENGING YET REALISTIC

Some people get fired up by goals that seem far-fetched; they rise to the occasion and perform extraordinarily well, says sports psychologist Robert Weinberg. "But others will give up. They'll say, 'You must be kidding!'"

In one study, researchers gave their subjects a seemingly impossible goal: to improve their sit-up performance by sixty repetitions over three months. Thirty percent of the subjects actually met the goal. Others, however, became demoralized and lost their motivation to train.

Figure out what type of goals work best for your personality. Research shows that moderately difficult goals — those that are challenging but within your capabilities—seem to work well for most people. If you don't reach high, you'll never know what you're capable of.

SET BOTH LONG-TERM AND SHORT-TERM GOALS

"I have two objectives that I operate from: the short-term goals and the 'things I need to do before I die' list," says ultramarathoner Tim Twietmeyer, five-time winner of the grueling 100-mile Western States Endurance Run. "The short-term goals drive what I do day to day, and the other list drives my planning for bigger, more outrageous efforts that I want to complete."

Even if you feel your life would be complete without snowshoeing for 26 hours over the Sierra Nevada Mountains—as Twietmeyer and some buddies recently did, becoming the first to cross the Sierra on foot since the 1850s—his general philosophy is a wise one.

Long-term goals, such as running a marathon or completing a cycling tour of Tuscany, will get your juices flowing, but you also need to establish steppingstones along the way. These more immediate goals will make your dream goals seem more achievable. Stacy Dragila, the world's first Olympic gold medalist in the women's pole vault, vividly remembers the day several years ago when her coach suggested she aim to vault 14 feet. "I thought, 'He's crazy! I'm only jumping 12' 6". How can I jump 14 feet?' But then he broke it down to daily and weekly goals, and it seemed doable." Dragila now holds the world record at 15' 9.25" and has her sights on 16 feet.

FOCUS ON A FEW GOALS

Don't set too many targets. Sure, we should all strive to eat more fiber, less saturated fat, more vegetables and fruits, less sugar, more whole grains, smaller portions, and so on and so on. But anyone who tries to achieve all of these objectives at once will go bonkers. For each general category—cardiovascular exercise, strength training, mind-body exercise, and nutrition—pick just one or two long-term goals and keep your

6

short-term goals manageable, too. For example, if your long-term nutrition goal is to cut way back on added sugar, your goal in the short run could be to drink water instead of soda when you go out to eat.

Chances are, if you do what it takes to achieve one or two goals, the rest will fall into place. For instance, if you simply aim to eat more fruits and vegetables, you'll automatically be eating more fiber and less saturated fat. Assess your priorities and focus on reaching the goals that are most important to you at any given time. If your big cardio goal is to train for a 10k race, maybe your mind-body goal could be simply to keep doing yoga once a week or stretch for three minutes a day.

FOCUS ON "PROCESS" RATHER THAN "OUTCOME" GOALS

This is just sports-psychology jargon for saying that you should focus on things you can control rather than those you can't. For example, even if you are determined to slim down, don't write in your log "My goal is to lose twelve pounds in eight weeks." That objective may be concrete and measurable—and it may even be realistic—but it's not necessarily within your control, since everyone's body works differently. Even if two overweight people eat and exercise exactly the same, they're not going to lose precisely the same amount of weight; some bodies just hang on to calories more easily than others.

By picking goals outside of your control, you may be setting yourself up for disappointment. Instead, choose objectives such as "lift weights three days a week" or "compete in two 5ks." Even if some of your goals are connected to a specific outcome, like completing a two-day breast-cancer walkathon or finishing in the top ten in a bike race, be sure to have back-up goals you can feel good about accomplishing in case something gets in the way of achieving your dream goals.

DEVELOP STRATEGIES TO ACHIEVE YOUR GOALS

Setting goals is key, but you also need a plan to get you to your destination. Completing an Olympic-distance triathlon might be well within your abilities, but if you don't know how to split your workout time among running, biking, and swimming or if you're unsure what intensity level to train at, you may not get the results you're looking for. Whether your goals are modest or lofty, consider hiring a trainer or coach to help you devise a plan. Also, there are countless training books and online workout and coaching programs to choose from. The books and Web sites in the Resources section can help you get started.

Even the simplest goals require some basic strategizing. For example, if you're aiming to exercise four days a week, examine the obstacles that have hindered you in the past and make some changes, whether it means hiring a babysitter, joining a gym closer to home, or waking up a half hour earlier.

PERIODICALLY EVALUATE YOUR GOALS

Whatever goals you set, don't be a slave to them. If your training isn't going according to plan — if you get injured or sidetracked by a major work project or if you're just not performing as well as you'd expected — cut yourself some slack. Cross out the old goals and pencil in new ones. "Goals are not etched in concrete," says legendary miler Steve Scott. "You have to be willing to be flexible and change your goals if things pop up."

You also have to be willing to be satisfied with your best effort, no matter what results it brings. Pole vaulter Stacy Dragila sets her sights as high as they come, but she keeps things in perspective as well. "You have to be realistic with yourself," she says. "You can have your 'dream, dream goals,' but also be satisfied with something a step lower than that."

Filling in Your Log

This is *your* log; you can make as many, or as few, notes as you want. The amount of information you track probably will vary over time. You may go through phases when you want to record every aspect of your exercise program, from your resting heart rate, to what you ate before each workout, to what the weather was like. At other times, you may simply want to write "Went for a swim."

Even if you record minimal information, it's a good idea to write *something* every day — including days you don't exercise. This way, when you look back you'll be able to distinguish between days you rested and days you were sick or injured. You'll have more information about how much training your body can handle.

When deciding what type of notes to make in your log, consider the experience of Matt Giusto, an Olympian in the 5,000-meter run. "I used to put way too much information in my log," he says. "I'd even write down which of my five pairs of shoes I wore, and track how much mileage I put on each shoe." Eventually he found the note-taking tedious and stopped recording his workouts altogether. "I figured I'd been doing it for so long that I could just rely on my common sense."

But abandoning his log wasn't the solution, either. "I'd get to a race and think, 'Wait, how did I train last year? How many rest days did I take?'" Now, Giusto has found a happy medium, logging how far he ran, how fast he ran, and how he felt. "I keep it simple," he says. "But it's helpful to have my log going again." Even if you have goals that are much more modest than those of a world-class athlete, figure out what level of record keeping works for you. Some people thrive on minutiae; others are more partial to the broad strokes.

Here's a rundown of the different sections of this log, along with several sample ways of recording your workouts. Eventually, you'll create your own shorthand system.

GOALS FOR THE NEXT SIX MONTHS

The goals page on the inside cover of the book is the place to consider the big picture: where you stand now and what you'd like to accomplish over the next six months. In the first section, you'll note your overall "dream goals," along with back-up goals.

Of course, it's tough to pinpoint a destination and devise a plan to get there if you're not clear on where you're starting from. Each of the subsequent sections — Cardio Exercise, Strength Training, Mind-Body Exercise, and Nutrition — is divided into Starting Point and Goals. Use the Starting Point space to record any details about your current abilities, your eating habits, relevant body measurements, and even your feelings about working out. When setting your goals, refer to the tips in the goals section.

For example, in the Cardio Exercise section, you might write:

Cardio Exercise

starting point Best 5k: 22:10; can run up Westridge Hill in 12:25; resting heart rate: 58; hate running hills!

goals Run 5k in 21:20; break 12 on Westridge; join a track club; stop hating hills so much.

GOALS FOR THE WEEK

Each Monday, you'll find a few lines where you can fill in your weekly goals.

You can set your weekly goals in a variety of ways. For instance, you can plan in terms of distance ("Bike 30 miles"), time ("Walk 40 minutes a day"), or number of sessions ("Lift weights three times" or "Take two yoga classes").

Although it's important to set concrete targets, keep in mind that not all goals need to involve numbers. You might aim to focus more on your Pilates technique, become a more skilled descender on your mountain bike, or just enjoy your workouts more. If you plan to push yourself hard some weeks, be sure to balance out your program with weeks of easy workouts, too. Many athletes schedule three successively more challenging weeks followed by a low-intensity, low-volume week.

MORNING INFO

This small section is deliberately vague. You can use it to note how many hours you slept, how soundly you snoozed, or simply how you felt, physically or emotionally, when you woke up.

You can also note your resting heart rate—the number of beats per minute that your heart beats when you're lying still. Taking your pulse first thing in the morning, either with a heart-rate monitor or by holding two fingers on your wrist, can be a good indication of how rested you are. If your heart rate is unusually elevated, this may be an indication that you're overtrained or haven't recovered from the previous day's workout and need a day of rest.

Tracking your resting heart rate over time also can give you an indication of how your fitness is improving. As you become more fit, your resting heart rate generally drops. Top endurance athletes have resting heart rates as low as 30 beats per minute, whereas a couch potato may have a resting heart rate of 80 beats per minute; in other words, an inactive person's heart may have to work more than twice as hard as an elite athlete's to pump the same amount of blood . But remember that your heart rate is in part genetically determined. If your resting heart rate is 60 and your training partner's is 52, this doesn't necessarily mean that your friend is in better shape. Don't compare your resting heart rate to anyone else's; instead, compare it to your own resting heart rate as you become more fit.

Many exercisers keep a heart-rate monitor on their nightstand so they can easily get a reading in the morning before they start moving around. For more details about measuring your heart rate, check out www.heartzones.com or www.trainingbible.com.

DAILY RATING

Although this box is at the top of the page, fill it out at the end of your workout. The Daily Rating is a measure of your intensity, not your success. Rate your workouts on a scale from 1 to 5 — in terms of how hard you pushed your body, not how far you went or how many calories you burned. A 1 rating would be a super-easy day; a 5 would be a killer workout. Shoot for a healthy mix of numbers. Log a "0" for days you don't exercise.

Each week, transfer your daily ratings to the chart on page 215 titled "Workout Ratings: The Big Picture." A glance at this chart will give you insight into your training. You might notice, for instance, that it's been two weeks since you took a day off or did a workout rated lower than 3 — maybe that's why you're feeling so wiped out. Or maybe it's been two weeks since you exercised at all!

CARDIO EXERCISE

In this section, you can record up to three different activities, including the amount of time you exercised, the distance you covered, and the intensity at which you worked out. There's also room to record additional aspects of your workout, such as how you felt, your workout partners, and the weather.

Say you used the elliptical trainer for 20 minutes on level 7, and it felt easy. Then you jogged on the treadmill for 20 minutes at 5.5 mph at a 1.0 incline and pushed hard. You might write:

elliptical	20 min., L7	easy
treadmill	20 min., 5.5, 1.0 inc.	pushed!

If you cycled 30 miles with your bike club on the coastal route, averaged 16.8 mph and felt especially strong on the hills, you might write:

Club ride, coast	30 mi./16.8 ave.	climbing strong!

STRENGTH TRAINING

In this section you can record your strength-training exercises, including how much weight you lifted and the number of sets and repetitions you performed. If you're a beginner, it's especially helpful to write down the names of the exercises. Many novices learn how to perform a routine without knowing which muscles each move is intended to strengthen. Writing "lat pulldown" will reinforce the notion that the exercise strengthens your back muscles. If you don't know the name of a particular exercise, ask a trainer at your gym or look it up in any of the strength-training books listed in the Resources section.

If you did 2 sets of lat pulldowns with 12 pounds, performing 8 reps per set, you might write:

lat pulldowns	12	2	8

Say you performed 3 sets of squats: The first set you did 12 reps with 75 pounds, the second, 10 reps with 90 pounds. On the third set, you used 105 pounds and struggled to eke out 7 reps. You might write:

squats	75, 90, 105	312, 10, 5	struggled on last

MIND-BODY WORKOUT

This box is new to the third edition. You can use it to record that you stretched, or even to identify the stretches you did. Or you can fill it with notes about Pilates, yoga, tai chi, or any other type of workout that doesn't directly fit the cardio or strength sections. The term "mind-body exercise" simply refers to any type of exercise that requires a conscious effort to link how you're feeling to what your body is doing.

NUTRITION NOTES

You can use this box to monitor your eating habits in countless ways. Just keep in mind that this log is not intended as a food diary. (There are plenty of other books designed for that purpose.) Rather than record every morsel you swallow, try focusing on one or two nutrition goals at a time. For instance, record how many vegetable servings you ate in a day, or note when you made a particularly nutritious food choice, such as "Ate turkey sandwich instead of Big Mac." You could record your breakfast choices for a week straight with the goal of maximizing your fiber intake and cutting back on bacon and cheese or sugary cereals. For a nutrient breakdown of just about any food, go to the U.S. Department of Agriculture's National Nutrient Database for Standard Reference, www.nal.usda.gov/fnic/foodcomp/search/.

To see how your eating habits affect your exercise performance, you might want to record what you eat before your workout. Over the course of a few weeks, look for any patterns. Maybe you tend to finish stronger on a two-hour bike ride when you eat a bagel with peanut butter than when you eat a plain bagel. Or maybe you perform better when you eat thirty minutes before a basketball game than if you eat two hours before.

DAILY WRAP-UP

This is a bonus section new to the third edition. Several readers requested a space for personal notes unrelated to exercise, sort of a "mental health" journal—a place to check in with yourself, monitor your stress level, your emotions, and other aspects of life that affect your general sense of well-being. Of course, you can also use it to make more extensive notes about your workouts or eating habits, schedule important meetings, even remind yourself to set your TiVo. The space is yours!

WEEKLY WRAP-UP

Here's your chance to look back at the week you just completed. Recording how much you accomplished one week will get you psyched as you start the next.

➡ Weekly Rating: This needn't be a precise average of your daily ratings, but use this 1-to-5 scale to record how hard you pushed your body during the week. Transfer your weekly ratings to the chart on page 215.

➡ Highlight of the Week: Use this line to note one specific accomplishment. It can be anything from "Survived kickboxing" to "Took a day off when I felt a cold coming on." There's a chart in the back of the log (page 216) to record significant personal bests.

➡ Goals: It's easy to set goals, but it's even easier to forget you ever did. This section will keep you honest, nudging you to look back at the goals you set the previous Monday. If you consistently fall short, perhaps you have unrealistic expectations; make a note about why you think you didn't meet your goals. On the other hand, if you frequently exceed your goals, perhaps you need more of a challenge.

➡ Cardio Notes: Assess your week as a whole, and record whether you felt strong or not up to par. You can use the boxes to record how many days of the week you did cardio exercise, the total number of hours you spent working out, and, depending on your activity, your total mileage or swim yardage. Don't feel compelled to use all three boxes; not all of them are relevant for every exerciser.

➡ Strength Notes: Jot down anything significant that happened on the weight-training front. In the "Total Sessions" space, note how many times you lifted weights. If you do a split routine (working different muscles on different days), you may want to use the space below to record how many days you worked each muscle group or body area. For instance, if you did two upper body workouts but worked your legs only once, you might note "upper: 2, lower: 1."

➡ Mind-Body Notes: Flip back through the week and note how many times you stretched or did yoga or Pilates, along with any feelings about the sessions or notes about your progress.

➡ Nutrition Notes: Record any patterns in your eating habits over the week. Maybe you chose nutritious snacks all week. Maybe you ate breakfast consistently or snacked on apples and peanut butter rather than your usual candy bar. Write it down!

Workout Diary

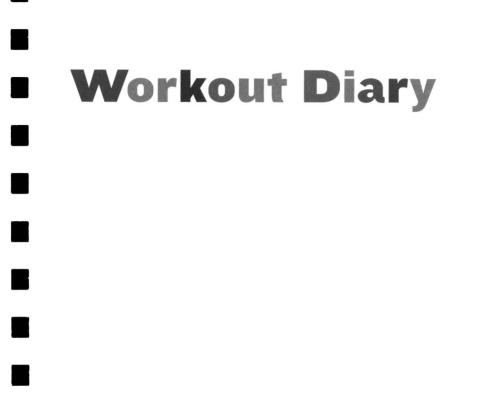

WEEK 1

Goals: _____

_____

_____

Dates: _____

MONDAY

MORNING INFO ☐ DAILY RATING ☐

CARDIO EXERCISE	TIME/DISTANCE/INTENSITY	NOTES
_____	_____	_____
_____	_____	_____
_____	_____	_____

STRENGTH TRAINING	WT.	SETS	REPS	NOTES
_____				_____
_____				_____
_____				_____
_____				_____
_____				_____
_____				_____
_____				_____
_____				_____
_____				_____

MIND-BODY NOTES

DAILY WRAP-UP

NUTRITION NOTES

_____

_____

_____

_____

MYTH BUSTER **Myth:** Exercising close to bedtime will keep you awake. **Reality:** There's no hard evidence that late-night workouts hinder sleep. In one study, men who cycled for 3 hours just 30 minutes before bedtime fell asleep as quickly as usual.

TUESDAY

MORNING INFO		DAILY RATING	

CARDIO EXERCISE	TIME/DISTANCE/INTENSITY	NOTES
_____	_____	_____
_____	_____	_____
_____	_____	_____
_____	_____	_____

STRENGTH TRAINING	WT.	SETS	REPS	NOTES
_____				_____
_____				_____
_____				_____
_____				_____
_____				_____
_____				_____
_____				_____
_____				_____
_____				_____

MIND-BODY NOTES

DAILY WRAP-UP

NUTRITION NOTES
_____
_____
_____
_____

NUTRITION NUGGET Tub margarines have less heart-damaging fat than stick margarines and butter. To choose the healthiest spread, look at the combined total of saturated fat and trans fat on the label, and go with the lowest number.

WEDNESDAY

MORNING INFO [ ]   DAILY RATING [ ]

CARDIO EXERCISE	TIME/DISTANCE/INTENSITY	NOTES
_____	_____	_____
_____	_____	_____
_____	_____	_____

STRENGTH TRAINING	WT.	SETS	REPS	NOTES
_____				_____
_____				_____
_____				_____
_____				_____
_____				_____
_____				_____
_____				_____
_____				_____
_____				_____

MIND-BODY NOTES

DAILY WRAP-UP

NUTRITION NOTES

BY THE NUMBERS **90:** Age of Abe Weintraub in 2000 when he finished the New York City Marathon in 7:25:12, the fastest ever time for a 90-year-old. **80:** Weintraub's age when he started competing.

THURSDAY

MORNING INFO		DAILY RATING	

CARDIO EXERCISE	TIME/DISTANCE/INTENSITY	NOTES

STRENGTH TRAINING	WT.	SETS	REPS	NOTES

MIND-BODY NOTES

DAILY WRAP-UP

NUTRITION NOTES

RESEARCH REPORT Pumping iron may be as good for your heart as it is for your muscles. In one study, men who lifted weights at least 30 minutes a week had a 23 percent lower heart-disease risk than men who didn't lift.

FRIDAY

MORNING INFO

DAILY RATING

CARDIO EXERCISE	TIME/DISTANCE/INTENSITY	NOTES

STRENGTH TRAINING	WT.	SETS	REPS	NOTES

MIND-BODY NOTES

DAILY WRAP-UP

NUTRITION NOTES

SATURDAY

MORNING INFO ☐

DAILY RATING ☐

CARDIO EXERCISE	TIME/DISTANCE/INTENSITY	NOTES
_____	_____	_____
_____	_____	_____
_____	_____	_____

STRENGTH TRAINING	WT.	SETS	REPS	NOTES
_____				_____
_____				_____
_____				_____
_____				_____
_____				_____
_____				_____
_____				_____
_____				_____

MIND-BODY NOTES

DAILY WRAP-UP

NUTRITION NOTES

_____

_____

_____

_____

TRAINING TRIVIA The word **gymnasium** comes from the Greek root **gymnos**, meaning "nude"; the literal meaning of gymnasium is "school for naked exercise."

SUNDAY

MORNING INFO ☐   DAILY RATING ☐

CARDIO EXERCISE	TIME/DISTANCE/INTENSITY	NOTES
_____	_____	_____
_____	_____	_____
_____	_____	_____

STRENGTH TRAINING	WT.	SETS	REPS	NOTES
_____				_____
_____				_____
_____				_____
_____				_____
_____				_____
_____				_____
_____				_____
_____				_____
_____				_____

MIND-BODY NOTES

DAILY WRAP-UP

NUTRITION NOTES
_____
_____
_____
_____

"You have to dream a little. If you stay in your comfort zone, you're not going to do anything special." **— DEENA KASTOR**, bronze medalist, marathon, 2004 Olympics

WEEKLY WRAP-UP

WEEKLY RATING ☐

Goals: MET _____ EXCEEDED _____ MAYBE NEXT WEEK _____

HIGHLIGHT OF THE WEEK _____

CARDIO NOTES   TOTAL SESSIONS ☐   MILES/ YARDS ☐   TOTAL HOURS ☐

_____

_____

_____

_____

_____

STRENGTH NOTES   TOTAL SESSIONS ☐

_____

_____

_____

_____

MIND-BODY NOTES

THOUGHTS ABOUT THE WEEK

NUTRITION NOTES _____

_____

_____

_____

WEEK 2

Goals:

Dates:

MONDAY

MORNING INFO

DAILY RATING

CARDIO EXERCISE	TIME/DISTANCE/INTENSITY	NOTES

STRENGTH TRAINING	WT.	SETS	REPS	NOTES

MIND-BODY NOTES

DAILY WRAP-UP

NUTRITION NOTES

MYTH BUSTER **Myth:** Adults should drink eight glasses of water a day. **Reality:** Although staying hydrated is important for performing your best, studies show that thirst is a reliable gauge of fluid requirements, so you needn't count glasses of water.

TUESDAY

MORNING INFO

DAILY RATING

CARDIO EXERCISE	TIME/DISTANCE/INTENSITY	NOTES

STRENGTH TRAINING	WT.	SETS	REPS	NOTES

MIND-BODY NOTES

DAILY WRAP-UP

NUTRITION NOTES

NUTRITION NUGGET Don't take food-label calorie counts literally. Federal law allows most products a 20 percent variance, so a cookie that supposedly contains 300 calories may actually contain 360 calories.

WEDNESDAY

MORNING INFO

DAILY RATING

CARDIO EXERCISE	TIME/DISTANCE/INTENSITY	NOTES

STRENGTH TRAINING	WT.	SETS	REPS	NOTES

MIND-BODY NOTES

DAILY WRAP-UP

NUTRITION NOTES

BY THE NUMBERS **50 mph:** Top speed of a lion. **32 mph:** Top speed of a giraffe. **30 mph:** Top speed of a kangaroo. **27.9 mph:** Top speed of a human. **25 mph:** Top speed of an elephant.

THURSDAY

MORNING INFO ☐ DAILY RATING ☐

CARDIO EXERCISE	TIME/DISTANCE/INTENSITY	NOTES
_____	_____	_____
_____	_____	_____
_____	_____	_____

STRENGTH TRAINING	WT.	SETS	REPS	NOTES
_____				_____
_____				_____
_____				_____
_____				_____
_____				_____
_____				_____
_____				_____
_____				_____
_____				_____

MIND-BODY NOTES

DAILY WRAP-UP

NUTRITION NOTES

RESEARCH REPORT We may burn 500 to 1,000 fewer calories per day than our ancestors, according to Australian researchers who paid actors to live at a nineteenth-century theme park, then compared their activity levels to those of office workers.

FRIDAY

MORNING
INFO

DAILY
RATING

CARDIO EXERCISE	TIME/DISTANCE/INTENSITY	NOTES

STRENGTH TRAINING	WT.	SETS	REPS	NOTES

MIND-BODY NOTES

DAILY WRAP-UP

NUTRITION NOTES

QUICK QUIZ Nutritionists recommend eating at least three servings of vegetables and two servings of fruit per day. How many Americans meet this ideal? **A)** 1 in 20 **B)** 1 in 11 **C)** 1 in 7 **D)** 1 in 4 (Answer on page 211.)

SATURDAY

MORNING INFO

DAILY RATING

CARDIO EXERCISE	TIME/DISTANCE/INTENSITY	NOTES

STRENGTH TRAINING	WT.	SETS	REPS	NOTES

MIND-BODY NOTES

DAILY WRAP-UP

NUTRITION NOTES

TRAINING TRIVIA Pilates machines were developed during World War I, when boxer Joseph Pilates was placed under forced internment in England with other German nationals. Pilates used bedsprings to create therapeutic exercises for the injured.

SUNDAY

MORNING INFO ▢

DAILY RATING ▢

CARDIO EXERCISE	TIME/DISTANCE/INTENSITY	NOTES

STRENGTH TRAINING	WT.	SETS	REPS	NOTES

MIND-BODY NOTES

DAILY WRAP-UP

NUTRITION NOTES

"I've learned to be thankful for each new day of training and to not let the hard times define my performances."
— **JEAN DRISCOLL**, eight-time Boston Marathon winner, wheelchair division; two-time Olympic silver medalist

WEEKLY WRAP-UP

WEEKLY RATING [ ]

Goals: MET _____ EXCEEDED _____ MAYBE NEXT WEEK _____

HIGHLIGHT OF THE WEEK _____

CARDIO NOTES   TOTAL SESSIONS [ ]   MILES/ YARDS [ ]   TOTAL HOURS [ ]

_____

_____

_____

_____

_____

STRENGTH NOTES   TOTAL SESSIONS [ ]

_____

_____

_____

_____

MIND-BODY NOTES

THOUGHTS ABOUT THE WEEK

NUTRITION NOTES _____

_____

_____

_____

_____

WEEK 3

Goals: _____

Dates: _____

MONDAY

MORNING INFO [ ]   DAILY RATING [ ]

CARDIO EXERCISE	TIME/DISTANCE/INTENSITY	NOTES
_____	_____	_____
_____	_____	_____
_____	_____	_____

STRENGTH TRAINING	WT.	SETS	REPS	NOTES
_____				_____
_____				_____
_____				_____
_____				_____
_____				_____
_____				_____
_____				_____
_____				_____
_____				_____
_____				_____

MIND-BODY NOTES

DAILY WRAP-UP

NUTRITION NOTES

MYTH BUSTER Myth: If you stop exercising, your muscle will turn to fat. **Reality:** Muscle can't turn into fat any more than it can turn into clam chowder. If you quit working out, your muscles will simply shrink and a greater proportion of your body weight will be fat.

TUESDAY

MORNING INFO

DAILY RATING

CARDIO EXERCISE	TIME/DISTANCE/INTENSITY	NOTES

STRENGTH TRAINING	WT.	SETS	REPS	NOTES

MIND-BODY NOTES

DAILY WRAP-UP

NUTRITION NOTES

NUTRITION NUGGET Eating fiber can help with weight control. Given permission to eat as much as they wanted, research subjects provided with high-fiber meals ate about 10 percent fewer calories than subjects served foods lower in fiber.

WEDNESDAY

MORNING INFO

DAILY RATING

CARDIO EXERCISE	TIME/DISTANCE/INTENSITY	NOTES

STRENGTH TRAINING	WT.	SETS	REPS	NOTES

MIND-BODY NOTES

DAILY WRAP-UP

NUTRITION NOTES

BY THE NUMBERS 135 miles: Distance of the Badwater Ultramarathon, often called the world's toughest footrace. 115° F: Average high temperature in Death Valley in July, when the race is held. 134° F: Record high in Death Valley in July.

THURSDAY

MORNING INFO ☐

DAILY RATING ☐

CARDIO EXERCISE	TIME/DISTANCE/INTENSITY	NOTES

STRENGTH TRAINING	WT.	SETS	REPS	NOTES

MIND-BODY NOTES

DAILY WRAP-UP

NUTRITION NOTES

RESEARCH REPORT Exercise can turn back the clock. In one study, postmenopausal women who lifted weights twice a week for a year had the strength and bone density levels of women 15 to 20 years younger.

FRIDAY

MORNING INFO

DAILY RATING

CARDIO EXERCISE	TIME/DISTANCE/INTENSITY	NOTES

STRENGTH TRAINING	WT.	SETS	REPS	NOTES

MIND-BODY NOTES

DAILY WRAP-UP

NUTRITION NOTES

QUICK QUIZ Which appetizer contains 3,000 calories and four days' worth of artery-clogging fat? **A)** cheese fries with ranch dressing **B)** batter-dipped fried whole onion plus dipping sauce **C)** twelve buffalo wings with bleu cheese dressing **D)** eight stuffed potato skins with sour cream (Answer on page 211.)

SATURDAY

MORNING INFO ☐   DAILY RATING ☐

CARDIO EXERCISE	TIME/DISTANCE/INTENSITY	NOTES
_____	_____	_____
_____	_____	_____
_____	_____	_____
_____		

STRENGTH TRAINING	WT.	SETS	REPS	NOTES
_____				_____
_____				_____
_____				_____
_____				_____
_____				_____
_____				_____
_____				_____
_____				_____
_____				_____
_____				_____

MIND-BODY NOTES

DAILY WRAP-UP

NUTRITION NOTES

_____
_____
_____
_____

TRAINING TRIVIA Swimming freestyle was unknown in Europe until 1844, when Native Americans used the stroke to beat the Brits in a London meet. Still, the Brits considered the splashing "grotesque" and continued to swim only breaststroke for several more decades.

SUNDAY

MORNING INFO ☐　　DAILY RATING ☐

CARDIO EXERCISE	TIME/DISTANCE/INTENSITY	NOTES
_____	_____	_____
_____	_____	_____
_____	_____	_____

STRENGTH TRAINING	WT.	SETS	REPS	NOTES
_____				_____
_____				_____
_____				_____
_____				_____
_____				_____
_____				_____
_____				_____
_____				_____
_____				_____
_____				

MIND-BODY NOTES

DAILY WRAP-UP

NUTRITION NOTES

> "As I've gotten older I listen to my body more, and I will allow a workout to possibly be too little rather than past the breaking point."
> — **AMY ACUFF**, four-time U.S. champion high jumper; three-time Olympian

WEEKLY WRAP-UP

WEEKLY RATING [ ]

Goals: MET _____ EXCEEDED _____ MAYBE NEXT WEEK _____

HIGHLIGHT OF THE WEEK _____

CARDIO NOTES   TOTAL SESSIONS [ ]   MILES/ YARDS [ ]   TOTAL HOURS [ ]

_____

_____

_____

_____

_____

STRENGTH NOTES   TOTAL SESSIONS [ ]

_____

_____

_____

_____

MIND-BODY NOTES

THOUGHTS ABOUT THE WEEK

NUTRITION NOTES _____

_____

_____

_____

_____

WEEK 4

Goals:

Dates:

MONDAY

CARDIO EXERCISE	TIME/DISTANCE/INTENSITY	NOTES

STRENGTH TRAINING	WT.	SETS	REPS	NOTES

MIND-BODY NOTES

DAILY WRAP-UP

NUTRITION NOTES

MYTH BUSTER **Myth:** Pedaling backward on the elliptical trainer works your butt and hamstrings better than pedaling forward. **Reality:** Pedaling backward offers no advantage. Like pedaling forward, it mainly works your quadriceps, but it also stresses your knees.

TUESDAY

MORNING INFO

DAILY RATING

CARDIO EXERCISE	TIME/DISTANCE/INTENSITY	NOTES

STRENGTH TRAINING	WT.	SETS	REPS	NOTES

MIND-BODY NOTES

DAILY WRAP-UP

NUTRITION NOTES

NUTRITION NUGGET Like saturated fat, trans fat — found in fried foods and processed baked goods — increases **LDL** cholesterol (the "bad" kind), escalating heart-attack and stroke risk. Worse, trans fat lowers **HDL** cholesterol, the type that helps keep arteries clean.

WEDNESDAY

MORNING INFO

DAILY RATING

CARDIO EXERCISE	TIME/DISTANCE/INTENSITY	NOTES

STRENGTH TRAINING	WT.	SETS	REPS	NOTES

MIND-BODY NOTES

DAILY WRAP-UP

NUTRITION NOTES

BY THE NUMBERS **35.7:** Percentage of Oregon residents who report exercising regularly, the highest rate of any state in the country. **16:** Percentage of Washington, D.C., residents who report working out regularly, the lowest nationwide.

THURSDAY

MORNING INFO ☐   DAILY RATING ☐

CARDIO EXERCISE	TIME/DISTANCE/INTENSITY	NOTES
_____	_____	_____
_____	_____	_____
_____	_____	_____
_____		_____

STRENGTH TRAINING	WT.	SETS	REPS	NOTES
_____				_____
_____				_____
_____				_____
_____				_____
_____				_____
_____				_____
_____				_____
_____				_____
_____				_____

MIND-BODY NOTES

DAILY WRAP-UP

NUTRITION NOTES
_____
_____
_____
_____

RESEARCH REPORT Fit women who train during and after pregnancy may end up with an even greater aerobic capacity than before, probably due to the increase in blood volume and changing hormone levels.

FRIDAY

MORNING INFO

DAILY RATING

CARDIO EXERCISE	TIME/DISTANCE/INTENSITY	NOTES

STRENGTH TRAINING	WT.	SETS	REPS	NOTES

MIND-BODY NOTES

DAILY WRAP-UP

NUTRITION NOTES

SATURDAY

MORNING
INFO

DAILY
RATING

CARDIO EXERCISE	TIME/DISTANCE/INTENSITY	NOTES

STRENGTH TRAINING	WT.	SETS	REPS	NOTES

MIND-BODY NOTES

DAILY WRAP-UP

NUTRITION NOTES

TRAINING TRIVIA At the 1896 Olympics in Athens, a woman defied the rules and ran the marathon course, prompting the event's founder to say, "No matter how toughened a sportswoman may be, her organism is not cut out to sustain certain shocks."

SUNDAY

MORNING INFO

DAILY RATING

CARDIO EXERCISE	TIME/DISTANCE/INTENSITY	NOTES

STRENGTH TRAINING	WT.	SETS	REPS	NOTES

MIND-BODY NOTES

DAILY WRAP-UP

NUTRITION NOTES

"Laugh at your foibles, celebrate every step of your progress, and measure your success by how much fun you're having, not by how many medals you win." — **JAYNE WILLIAMS**, author, **Slow Fat Triathlete**

WEEKLY WRAP-UP

WEEKLY RATING [ ]

Goals: MET _____ EXCEEDED _____ MAYBE NEXT WEEK _____

HIGHLIGHT OF THE WEEK _____

CARDIO NOTES   TOTAL SESSIONS [ ]   MILES/ YARDS [ ]   TOTAL HOURS [ ]

_____

_____

_____

_____

_____

STRENGTH NOTES   TOTAL SESSIONS [ ]

_____

_____

_____

_____

MIND-BODY NOTES	THOUGHTS ABOUT THE WEEK

NUTRITION NOTES _____

_____

_____

_____

_____

WEEK 5

Goals:

Dates:

MONDAY

MORNING INFO

DAILY RATING

CARDIO EXERCISE

TIME/DISTANCE/INTENSITY

NOTES

STRENGTH TRAINING

	WT.	SETS	REPS	NOTES

MIND-BODY NOTES

DAILY WRAP-UP

NUTRITION NOTES

MYTH BUSTER **Myth:** You burn more calories exercising in the cold. **Reality:** You burn about the same number of calories regardless of the weather, unless you're so cold your teeth are chattering, in which case you do burn more calories but risk hypothermia.

TUESDAY

MORNING INFO [   ] DAILY RATING [   ]

CARDIO EXERCISE	TIME/DISTANCE/INTENSITY	NOTES

STRENGTH TRAINING	WT.	SETS	REPS	NOTES

MIND-BODY NOTES

DAILY WRAP-UP

NUTRITION NOTES

NUTRITION NUGGET Americans get only half the recommended 25 to 38 grams of fiber daily. To boost your intake, choose whole fruits over juices. A six-ounce serving of apple juice contains 90 calories and only .2 grams of fiber; an apple contains 72 calories and 2.5 grams of fiber.

WEDNESDAY

MORNING INFO [ ]

DAILY RATING [ ]

CARDIO EXERCISE	TIME/DISTANCE/INTENSITY	NOTES
_____	_____	_____
_____	_____	_____
_____	_____	_____

STRENGTH TRAINING	WT.	SETS	REPS	NOTES
_____				_____
_____				_____
_____				_____
_____				_____
_____				_____
_____				_____
_____				_____
_____				_____
_____				_____

MIND-BODY NOTES

DAILY WRAP-UP

NUTRITION NOTES

_____

_____

_____

_____

BY THE NUMBERS **17:31:** Time in the 1.5-mile run required by the Honolulu Police Department. **14:52:** Time required by the Ohio County Sheriff's Department. **13 minutes:** Time required by women in the British Air Force. **11 minutes:** Time required by men in the British Air Force.

THURSDAY

MORNING INFO ▢   DAILY RATING ▢

CARDIO EXERCISE	TIME/DISTANCE/INTENSITY	NOTES

STRENGTH TRAINING	WT.	SETS	REPS	NOTES

MIND-BODY NOTES

DAILY WRAP-UP

NUTRITION NOTES

RESEARCH REPORT Multiple short bouts of exercise are just as effective for fitness and weight loss as one long session. In one study, subjects who exercised for three 10-minute sessions a day reaped the same benefits as subjects who exercised for one 30-minute session.

FRIDAY

MORNING INFO

DAILY RATING

CARDIO EXERCISE	TIME/DISTANCE/INTENSITY	NOTES

STRENGTH TRAINING	WT.	SETS	REPS	NOTES

MIND-BODY NOTES

DAILY WRAP-UP

NUTRITION NOTES

QUICK QUIZ Which cut of meat has the most saturated fat per four-ounce, choice-grade serving? **A)** porterhouse steak **B)** steak-broiled top sirloin **C)** roasted eye of round **D)** braised shortrib (Answer on page 211.)

SATURDAY

MORNING INFO

DAILY RATING

CARDIO EXERCISE	TIME/DISTANCE/INTENSITY	NOTES

STRENGTH TRAINING	WT.	SETS	REPS	NOTES

MIND-BODY NOTES

DAILY WRAP-UP

NUTRITION NOTES

TRAINING TRIVIA Historians speculate that dumbbells got their name because early weights were bell-shaped forms cast from the same molds used to make hand bells — but either poured solid or made without a tongue so they were "dumb."

SUNDAY

MORNING INFO ☐   DAILY RATING ☐

CARDIO EXERCISE	TIME/DISTANCE/INTENSITY	NOTES
_____	_____	_____
_____	_____	_____
_____	_____	_____

STRENGTH TRAINING	WT.	SETS	REPS	NOTES
_____				_____
_____				_____
_____				_____
_____				_____
_____				_____
_____				_____
_____				_____
_____				_____
_____				_____
_____				_____
_____				_____

MIND-BODY NOTES

DAILY WRAP-UP

NUTRITION NOTES

"What keeps me motivated is preparing for the next challenge. I always have something in my mind, whether it's a competition or a solo adventure." — **TIM TWIETMEYER**, five-time winner, 100-mile Western States Endurance Run

WEEKLY WRAP-UP

WEEKLY RATING ☐

Goals: MET _____ EXCEEDED _____ MAYBE NEXT WEEK _____

HIGHLIGHT OF THE WEEK _____

CARDIO NOTES   TOTAL SESSIONS ☐   MILES/ YARDS ☐   TOTAL HOURS ☐

_____

_____

_____

_____

_____

_____

STRENGTH NOTES   TOTAL SESSIONS ☐

_____

_____

_____

_____

_____

MIND-BODY NOTES	THOUGHTS ABOUT THE WEEK

NUTRITION NOTES _____

_____

_____

_____

_____

WEEK
6

Goals: _____

_____

_____

Dates: _____

MONDAY

MORNING INFO [   ]   DAILY RATING [   ]

CARDIO EXERCISE	TIME/DISTANCE/INTENSITY	NOTES
_____	_____	_____
_____	_____	_____
_____	_____	_____

STRENGTH TRAINING	WT.	SETS	REPS	NOTES
_____				_____
_____				_____
_____				_____
_____				_____
_____				_____
_____				_____
_____				_____
_____				_____
_____				_____
_____				_____

MIND-BODY NOTES

DAILY WRAP-UP

NUTRITION NOTES

_____

_____

_____

_____

MYTH BUSTER **Myth:** For every pound of muscle you build, your body burns 50 to 100 extra calories. **Reality:** Your body actually burns closer to 10 to 15 calories per pound of muscle. Lifting weights can boost your metabolism but isn't a magic bullet.

TUESDAY

MORNING INFO

DAILY RATING

CARDIO EXERCISE	TIME/DISTANCE/INTENSITY	NOTES
_____	_____	_____
_____	_____	_____
_____	_____	_____

STRENGTH TRAINING	WT.	SETS	REPS	NOTES
_____				_____
_____				_____
_____				_____
_____				_____
_____				_____
_____				_____
_____				_____
_____				_____
_____				_____
_____				_____

MIND-BODY NOTES

DAILY WRAP-UP

NUTRITION NOTES

NUTRITION NUGGET The 7-Eleven Double Gulp, a 64-ounce soda with nearly 800 calories, is ten times the size of a Coca-Cola when it was introduced in the fifties. Soda sizes have gotten so big that auto manufacturers have installed larger cup holders.

WEDNESDAY

MORNING INFO

DAILY RATING

CARDIO EXERCISE	TIME/DISTANCE/INTENSITY	NOTES

STRENGTH TRAINING	WT.	SETS	REPS	NOTES

MIND-BODY NOTES

DAILY WRAP-UP

NUTRITION NOTES

BY THE NUMBERS **38° F:** Temperature of the Bering Strait during the last half hour of Lynne Cox's famous two hour, seven minute crossing of the 2.7-mile stretch between Alaska and Russia. **33° F:** Temperature of the ocean when Cox swam 1.22 miles to Antarctica.

THURSDAY

MORNING INFO [   ]   DAILY RATING [   ]

CARDIO EXERCISE	TIME/DISTANCE/INTENSITY	NOTES

STRENGTH TRAINING	WT.	SETS	REPS	NOTES

MIND-BODY NOTES

DAILY WRAP-UP

NUTRITION NOTES

RESEARCH REPORT Working out in front of an audience may help you perform better. In one study, weight lifters were able to hoist five pounds more in front of spectators — even though the crowd was silent — than when they lifted alone.

FRIDAY

MORNING INFO

DAILY RATING

CARDIO EXERCISE	TIME/DISTANCE/INTENSITY	NOTES

STRENGTH TRAINING	WT.	SETS	REPS	NOTES

MIND-BODY NOTES

DAILY WRAP-UP

NUTRITION NOTES

QUICK QUIZ The government's serving size for spaghetti marinara is one cup, with 250 calories. A typical restaurant serving is A) two cups; 500 calories B) three cups; 750 calories C) three and a half cups; 875 calories D) four cups; 1,000 calories (Answer on page 211.)

SATURDAY

MORNING INFO		DAILY RATING	

CARDIO EXERCISE	TIME/DISTANCE/INTENSITY	NOTES

STRENGTH TRAINING	WT.	SETS	REPS	NOTES

MIND-BODY NOTES

DAILY WRAP-UP

NUTRITION NOTES

TRAINING TRIVIA Tennis was first played by medieval French monks, who hit the ball with their hands. For more cushioning, they began using webbed gloves. The ball was a wad of hair, wool, or cork wrapped in string and cloth or leather.

SUNDAY

MORNING INFO

DAILY RATING

CARDIO EXERCISE	TIME/DISTANCE/INTENSITY	NOTES

STRENGTH TRAINING	WT.	SETS	REPS	NOTES

MIND-BODY NOTES

DAILY WRAP-UP

NUTRITION NOTES

"You need to be flexible with your workouts. Some days you just don't have it, but some days you will shock yourself with your strength."
— **DOTSIE COWDEN**, U.S. National Cycling Team member

WEEKLY WRAP-UP

WEEKLY RATING

Goals: MET _____ EXCEEDED _____ MAYBE NEXT WEEK _____

HIGHLIGHT OF THE WEEK _____

CARDIO NOTES   TOTAL SESSIONS [ ]   MILES/ YARDS [ ]   TOTAL HOURS [ ]

_____

_____

_____

_____

_____

STRENGTH NOTES   TOTAL SESSIONS [ ]

_____

_____

_____

_____

MIND-BODY NOTES

THOUGHTS ABOUT THE WEEK

NUTRITION NOTES _____

_____

_____

_____

WEEK
7

Goals: _____
_____
_____

Dates: _____

MONDAY

MORNING INFO ☐ **DAILY RATING** ☐

CARDIO EXERCISE	TIME/DISTANCE/INTENSITY	NOTES
_____	_____	_____
_____	_____	_____
_____	_____	_____

STRENGTH TRAINING	WT.	SETS	REPS	NOTES
_____				_____
_____				_____
_____				_____
_____				_____
_____				_____
_____				_____
_____				_____
_____				_____
_____				_____

MIND-BODY NOTES

DAILY WRAP-UP

NUTRITION NOTES
_____
_____
_____

MYTH BUSTER **Myth:** For weight loss, it's always better to eat six small meals a day than three large ones. **Reality:** Frequent eating doesn't necessarily translate into better calorie control. Some people may eat more food if given the chance to eat more often.

TUESDAY

MORNING INFO ☐

DAILY RATING ☐

CARDIO EXERCISE	TIME/DISTANCE/INTENSITY	NOTES
_____	_____	_____
_____	_____	_____
_____	_____	_____

STRENGTH TRAINING	WT.	SETS	REPS	NOTES
_____				_____
_____				_____
_____				_____
_____				_____
_____				_____
_____				_____
_____				_____
_____				_____
_____				_____

MIND-BODY NOTES

DAILY WRAP-UP

NUTRITION NOTES
_____
_____
_____
_____

NUTRITION NUGGET The advantages of low-carb diets appear to be small and short-lived. In a one-year study, low-carb dieters began regaining weight after six months and at one year were no better off than low-fat dieters. Both groups had high dropout rates.

WEDNESDAY

MORNING INFO

DAILY RATING

CARDIO EXERCISE	TIME/DISTANCE/INTENSITY	NOTES

STRENGTH TRAINING	WT.	SETS	REPS	NOTES

MIND-BODY NOTES

DAILY WRAP-UP

NUTRITION NOTES

BY THE NUMBERS $500 million: Estimated amount that physically active Americans save the country yearly in health-care costs. $75 billion: Estimated cost of inactivity. 9.4: Percentage of national health expenditures associated with inactivity and obesity.

THURSDAY

MORNING INFO

DAILY RATING

CARDIO EXERCISE	TIME/DISTANCE/INTENSITY	NOTES

STRENGTH TRAINING	WT.	SETS	REPS	NOTES

MIND-BODY NOTES

DAILY WRAP-UP

NUTRITION NOTES

RESEARCH REPORT Running can add years to your life. In a 13-year study, members of a 50-plus running club lived on average 2.3 years longer than their sedentary age-mates and delayed the onset of disability by nearly 9 years.

FRIDAY

MORNING INFO

DAILY RATING

CARDIO EXERCISE	TIME/DISTANCE/INTENSITY	NOTES

STRENGTH TRAINING	WT.	SETS	REPS	NOTES

MIND-BODY NOTES

DAILY WRAP-UP

NUTRITION NOTES

QUICK QUIZ How many calories will you save by forgoing the whipped cream on your blended coffee drink? **A)** 160 **B)** 100 **C)** 60 **D)** 30 (Answer on page 211.)

SATURDAY

MORNING INFO [ ]

DAILY RATING [ ]

CARDIO EXERCISE	TIME/DISTANCE/INTENSITY	NOTES
_____	_____	_____
_____	_____	_____
_____	_____	_____
_____	_____	_____

STRENGTH TRAINING	WT.	SETS	REPS	NOTES
_____				_____
_____				_____
_____				_____
_____				_____
_____				_____
_____				_____
_____				_____
_____				_____
_____				_____

MIND-BODY NOTES

DAILY WRAP-UP

NUTRITION NOTES _____

TRAINING TRIVIA Being a "trainer to the stars" is nothing new. In the early 1800s, exercise specialists were paid to train royalty, including King Edward of England, the Empress of Russia, and the Crown Prince of Norway.

SUNDAY

MORNING INFO ☐   DAILY RATING ☐

CARDIO EXERCISE	TIME/DISTANCE/INTENSITY	NOTES
_____	_____	_____
_____	_____	_____
_____	_____	_____

STRENGTH TRAINING	WT.	SETS	REPS	NOTES
_____				_____
_____				_____
_____				_____
_____				_____
_____				_____
_____				_____
_____				_____
_____				_____
_____				_____
_____				_____

MIND-BODY NOTES

DAILY WRAP-UP

NUTRITION NOTES

"Every player I play with or against can teach me something, so I try to watch and learn. When we think we know it all is when we stop growing and becoming better!" **— SHANNON MACMILLAN**, U.S. National Soccer Team member, 2000 Olympic silver medalist

WEEKLY WRAP-UP

WEEKLY RATING [ ]

Goals: MET _____ EXCEEDED _____ MAYBE NEXT WEEK _____

HIGHLIGHT OF THE WEEK _____

CARDIO NOTES   TOTAL SESSIONS [ ]   MILES/ YARDS [ ]   TOTAL HOURS [ ]

_____

_____

_____

_____

_____

STRENGTH NOTES   TOTAL SESSIONS [ ]

_____

_____

_____

_____

_____

MIND-BODY NOTES

THOUGHTS ABOUT THE WEEK

NUTRITION NOTES _____

WEEK 8

Goals: _____
_____
_____

Dates: _____

MONDAY

MORNING INFO		DAILY RATING	

CARDIO EXERCISE	TIME/DISTANCE/INTENSITY	NOTES
_____	_____	_____
_____	_____	_____
_____	_____	_____

STRENGTH TRAINING	WT.	SETS	REPS	NOTES
_____				_____
_____				_____
_____				_____
_____				_____
_____				_____
_____				_____
_____				_____
_____				_____
_____				_____

MIND-BODY NOTES

DAILY WRAP-UP

NUTRITION NOTES
_____
_____
_____

MYTH BUSTER Myth: Wearing a weight belt will help protect your back. **Reality:** Studies have found no difference in back pain between workers who wear belts and those who don't. The U.S. government doesn't recommend belts for workers involved in heavy lifting.

TUESDAY

MORNING INFO

DAILY RATING

CARDIO EXERCISE	TIME/DISTANCE/INTENSITY	NOTES

STRENGTH TRAINING	WT.	SETS	REPS	NOTES

MIND-BODY NOTES

DAILY WRAP-UP

NUTRITION NOTES

NUTRITION NUGGET Just because a food package features a picture of a particular fruit doesn't mean there's any of that fruit in the product. Those chewy bits of fruit in Quaker "Strawberries & Cream" Instant Oatmeal are actually dehydrated apples dyed red.

WEDNESDAY

MORNING INFO [   ]

DAILY RATING [   ]

CARDIO EXERCISE	TIME/DISTANCE/INTENSITY	NOTES

STRENGTH TRAINING	WT.	SETS	REPS	NOTES

MIND-BODY NOTES

DAILY WRAP-UP

NUTRITION NOTES

BY THE NUMBERS 4:46: The average per-mile pace of Paul Tergat when he broke the marathon world record in the 2003 Berlin Marathon with a time of 2:04:55. 7:12: Average per-mile pace of the 1896 Olympic marathon winner.

THURSDAY

MORNING INFO ☐   DAILY RATING ☐

CARDIO EXERCISE	TIME/DISTANCE/INTENSITY	NOTES

STRENGTH TRAINING	WT.	SETS	REPS	NOTES

MIND-BODY NOTES

DAILY WRAP-UP

NUTRITION NOTES

RESEARCH REPORT Regular exercise reduces the systolic (top number) and diastolic (bottom number) blood pressure by an average of seven to ten points. If you have high blood pressure, aim to exercise from 20 to 60 minutes, three to five times a week.

FRIDAY

MORNING INFO

DAILY RATING

CARDIO EXERCISE	TIME/DISTANCE/INTENSITY	NOTES

STRENGTH TRAINING	WT.	SETS	REPS	NOTES

MIND-BODY NOTES

DAILY WRAP-UP

NUTRITION NOTES

QUICK QUIZ Which of the following breads contain 0 grams of fiber per slice? **A)** Milbrook's Cracked Wheat Bread **B)** Oroweat 12 Grain Bread **C)** Wonder Bread **D)** Pepperidge Farm Very Thin Sliced Wheat (Answer on page 212.)

SATURDAY

MORNING INFO ☐

DAILY RATING ☐

CARDIO EXERCISE	TIME/DISTANCE/INTENSITY	NOTES

STRENGTH TRAINING	WT.	SETS	REPS	NOTES

MIND-BODY NOTES

DAILY WRAP-UP

NUTRITION NOTES

TRAINING TRIVIA In 1943 the government ordered swimsuit fabric reduced due to wartime shortages. The result: two-piece suits. Refined in Paris, the bikini was named for Bikini Atoll, a nuclear-weapons test site in the Pacific. The reasoning: The ensuing excitement would be like an atomic bomb.

SUNDAY

MORNING INFO ☐   DAILY RATING ☐

CARDIO EXERCISE	TIME/DISTANCE/INTENSITY	NOTES

STRENGTH TRAINING	WT.	SETS	REPS	NOTES

MIND-BODY NOTES

DAILY WRAP-UP

NUTRITION NOTES

"I just have to start putting on my running shoes and my dog Wasatch goes crazy. Seeing how much he wants to go for a run is all the inspiration I need." — **ANN TRASON**, 14-time winner, 100-mile Western States Endurance Run

WEEKLY WRAP-UP

WEEKLY RATING ☐

Goals: MET _____ EXCEEDED _____ MAYBE NEXT WEEK _____

HIGHLIGHT OF THE WEEK _____

CARDIO NOTES   TOTAL SESSIONS ☐   MILES/ YARDS ☐   TOTAL HOURS ☐

_____

_____

_____

_____

_____

STRENGTH NOTES   TOTAL SESSIONS ☐

_____

_____

_____

_____

MIND-BODY NOTES	THOUGHTS ABOUT THE WEEK

NUTRITION NOTES _____

_____

_____

_____

WEEK 9

Goals: _____

_____

_____

Dates: _____

MONDAY

MORNING INFO		DAILY RATING	

CARDIO EXERCISE	TIME/DISTANCE/INTENSITY	NOTES

STRENGTH TRAINING	WT.	SETS	REPS	NOTES

MIND-BODY NOTES

DAILY WRAP-UP

NUTRITION NOTES

MYTH BUSTER **Myth:** Water exercise is a poor calorie burner. **Reality:** Sprinting in chest-high water can burn as many as 17 calories per minute, the same as running at a 5-minute-mile pace. Deep-water running with a flotation belt can burn 13 to 15 calories per minute.

TUESDAY

MORNING INFO ☐ DAILY RATING ☐

CARDIO EXERCISE	TIME/DISTANCE/INTENSITY	NOTES
_____	_____	_____
_____	_____	_____
_____	_____	_____
_____	_____	_____

STRENGTH TRAINING	WT.	SETS	REPS	NOTES
_____				_____
_____				_____
_____				_____
_____				_____
_____				_____
_____				_____
_____				_____
_____				_____
_____				_____

MIND-BODY NOTES

DAILY WRAP-UP

NUTRITION NOTES

NUTRITION NUGGET Cereals sold at health-food markets may not be any more nutritious than cereals sold at the regular supermarket. Many organic brands contain no fiber and are not fortified with vitamins and minerals. Read the label.

WEDNESDAY

MORNING INFO

DAILY RATING

CARDIO EXERCISE	TIME/DISTANCE/INTENSITY	NOTES

STRENGTH TRAINING	WT.	SETS	REPS	NOTES

MIND-BODY NOTES

DAILY WRAP-UP

NUTRITION NOTES

BY THE NUMBERS **8,100:** Average daily calories burned by competitors during **22** days and **2,400** miles of the Tour de France. **342,000:** Approximate number of pedal strokes taken per rider during the race.

THURSDAY

MORNING INFO ☐

DAILY RATING ☐

CARDIO EXERCISE	TIME/DISTANCE/INTENSITY	NOTES

STRENGTH TRAINING	WT.	SETS	REPS	NOTES

MIND-BODY NOTES

DAILY WRAP-UP

NUTRITION NOTES

RESEARCH REPORT Physically active men and women may be 40 to 50 percent less likely to develop colon cancer than sedentary people. Active women may be 30 to 40 percent less likely to develop breast cancer.

FRIDAY

MORNING INFO

DAILY RATING

CARDIO EXERCISE	TIME/DISTANCE/INTENSITY	NOTES

STRENGTH TRAINING	WT.	SETS	REPS	NOTES

MIND-BODY NOTES

DAILY WRAP-UP

NUTRITION NOTES

QUICK QUIZ Which of the following fruits contains the most fiber? **A)** one medium apple **B)** one cup of blueberries **C)** one pear **D)** one banana (Answer on page 212.)

SATURDAY

MORNING INFO [ ]

DAILY RATING [ ]

CARDIO EXERCISE	TIME/DISTANCE/INTENSITY	NOTES
___	___	___
___	___	___
___	___	___

STRENGTH TRAINING	WT.	SETS	REPS	NOTES
___				___
___				___
___				___
___				___
___				___
___				___
___				___

MIND-BODY NOTES

DAILY WRAP-UP

NUTRITION NOTES

___

___

___

___

TRAINING TRIVIA A primitive version of the bicycle was invented in 1817 by a baron who wanted to get around the royal gardens faster. However, the device had no pedals and, being impractical for transportation, enjoyed only short-lived popularity.

SUNDAY

MORNING INFO

DAILY RATING

CARDIO EXERCISE	TIME/DISTANCE/INTENSITY	NOTES

STRENGTH TRAINING	WT.	SETS	REPS	NOTES

MIND-BODY NOTES

DAILY WRAP-UP

NUTRITION NOTES

"Eating poorly, partying too much, and getting little rest — it all catches up with you. It's important to take care of yourself off the track if you want to reap the rewards of a good training program."
— **DARVIS PATTON**, 2003 World Outdoor 200-meter champion

WEEKLY WRAP-UP

WEEKLY RATING ☐

Goals: MET _____ EXCEEDED _____ MAYBE NEXT WEEK _____

HIGHLIGHT OF THE WEEK _____

CARDIO NOTES   TOTAL SESSIONS ☐   MILES/YARDS ☐   TOTAL HOURS ☐

_____
_____
_____
_____
_____

STRENGTH NOTES   TOTAL SESSIONS ☐

_____
_____
_____
_____

MIND-BODY NOTES

THOUGHTS ABOUT THE WEEK

NUTRITION NOTES _____
_____
_____
_____
_____

WEEK 10

Goals: _____

_____

_____

Dates: _____

MONDAY

MORNING INFO [ ] **DAILY RATING** [ ]

CARDIO EXERCISE	TIME/DISTANCE/INTENSITY	NOTES
_____	_____	_____
_____	_____	_____
_____	_____	_____

STRENGTH TRAINING	WT.	SETS	REPS	NOTES
_____				_____
_____				_____
_____				_____
_____				_____
_____				_____
_____				_____
_____				_____
_____				_____
_____				_____
_____				_____

MIND-BODY NOTES

DAILY WRAP-UP

NUTRITION NOTES

_____

_____

_____

_____

MYTH BUSTER **Myth:** Lactic acid is responsible for the muscle soreness you feel a day or two after a hard workout. **Reality:** Most lactic acid is cleared out via blood circulation within 15 minutes to 1 hour after a workout. Soreness is caused by microscopic muscle tears.

TUESDAY

MORNING INFO ☐   DAILY RATING ☐

CARDIO EXERCISE	TIME/DISTANCE/INTENSITY	NOTES
_____	_____	_____
_____	_____	_____
_____	_____	_____

STRENGTH TRAINING	WT.	SETS	REPS	NOTES
_____				_____
_____				_____
_____				_____
_____				_____
_____				_____
_____				_____
_____				_____
_____				_____

MIND-BODY NOTES

DAILY WRAP-UP

NUTRITION NOTES
_____
_____
_____
_____

NUTRITION NUGGET The government allows manufacturers to round down trans fat numbers on food labels, so a food that actually contains 1.4 grams of trans fat will appear to contain 1 gram. Foods with less than .5 grams per serving can claim to be trans fat–free.

WEDNESDAY

MORNING INFO ☐

DAILY RATING ☐

CARDIO EXERCISE	TIME/DISTANCE/INTENSITY	NOTES

STRENGTH TRAINING	WT.	SETS	REPS	NOTES

MIND-BODY NOTES

DAILY WRAP-UP

NUTRITION NOTES

BY THE NUMBERS **5.2:** Number of boxing injuries per 1,000 "athlete exposures." **3.8:** Number of tackle football injuries per 1,000 exposures. **1.9:** Number of basketball injuries per 1,000 exposures. **.6:** Number of running injuries per 1,000 exposures.

THURSDAY

MORNING INFO ☐

DAILY RATING ☐

CARDIO EXERCISE	TIME/DISTANCE/INTENSITY	NOTES

STRENGTH TRAINING	WT.	SETS	REPS	NOTES

MIND-BODY NOTES

DAILY WRAP-UP

NUTRITION NOTES

RESEARCH REPORT For weight loss, exercise and dieting works better than dieting alone. One study found that groups who did aerobic exercise and cut calories lost on average 4.2 pounds more than dieters. Groups adding weight training lost an extra 2 pounds.

FRIDAY

MORNING INFO

DAILY RATING

CARDIO EXERCISE	TIME/DISTANCE/INTENSITY	NOTES

STRENGTH TRAINING	WT.	SETS	REPS	NOTES

MIND-BODY NOTES

DAILY WRAP-UP

NUTRITION NOTES

SATURDAY

MORNING INFO		DAILY RATING	

CARDIO EXERCISE   **TIME/DISTANCE/INTENSITY**   **NOTES**

_____   _____   _____

_____   _____   _____

_____   _____   _____

STRENGTH TRAINING   **WT.**   **SETS**   **REPS**   **NOTES**

MIND-BODY NOTES

DAILY WRAP-UP

NUTRITION NOTES

TRAINING TRIVIA The butterfly stroke, which evolved from the breaststroke, was developed in the 1930s, but it wasn't until the late 1950s that it was recognized as a separate stroke for competition.

SUNDAY

MORNING INFO

DAILY RATING

CARDIO EXERCISE	TIME/DISTANCE/INTENSITY	NOTES

STRENGTH TRAINING	WT.	SETS	REPS	NOTES

MIND-BODY NOTES

DAILY WRAP-UP

NUTRITION NOTES

"What keeps me motivated is my background. I have opportunities that many do not have in East Africa, where I was born, so I want to maximize my talent to the fullest." — **MEB KEFLEZIGHI**, silver medalist, marathon, 2004 Olympics

WEEKLY WRAP-UP

WEEKLY RATING [ ]

Goals: MET _____ EXCEEDED _____ MAYBE NEXT WEEK _____

HIGHLIGHT OF THE WEEK _____

CARDIO NOTES   TOTAL SESSIONS [ ]   MILES/ YARDS [ ]   TOTAL HOURS [ ]

_____

_____

_____

_____

_____

STRENGTH NOTES   TOTAL SESSIONS [ ]

_____

_____

_____

_____

MIND-BODY NOTES | THOUGHTS ABOUT THE WEEK

NUTRITION NOTES _____

_____

_____

_____

_____

WEEK 11

Goals:

_____

_____

_____

Dates: _____

MONDAY

MORNING INFO ☐   DAILY RATING ☐

CARDIO EXERCISE	TIME/DISTANCE/INTENSITY	NOTES
_____	_____	_____
_____	_____	_____
_____	_____	_____

STRENGTH TRAINING	WT.	SETS	REPS	NOTES
_____				_____
_____				_____
_____				_____
_____				_____
_____				_____
_____				_____
_____				_____
_____				_____
_____				_____

MIND-BODY NOTES

DAILY WRAP-UP

NUTRITION NOTES

_____

_____

_____

MYTH BUSTER **Myth:** Pilates will give you long, lean muscles. **Reality:** The length of your muscles is dictated by the length of your bones and the way your muscles attach to them. Though Pilates has great benefits, it can't make a shotputter look like a ballerina.

TUESDAY

MORNING INFO

DAILY RATING

CARDIO EXERCISE	TIME/DISTANCE/INTENSITY	NOTES

STRENGTH TRAINING	WT.	SETS	REPS	NOTES

MIND-BODY NOTES

DAILY WRAP-UP

NUTRITION NOTES

NUTRITION NUGGET The National Cancer Institute has identified about 35 plant foods and herbs with cancer-protective properties. Those with the highest anticancer activity include garlic, soybeans, cabbage, ginger, licorice root, carrots, celery, and parsley.

WEDNESDAY

MORNING INFO ☐

DAILY RATING ☐

CARDIO EXERCISE	TIME/DISTANCE/INTENSITY	NOTES
_____	_____	_____
_____	_____	_____
_____	_____	_____
_____	_____	_____

STRENGTH TRAINING	WT.	SETS	REPS	NOTES
_____				_____
_____				_____
_____				_____
_____				_____
_____				_____
_____				_____
_____				_____
_____				_____
_____				_____

MIND-BODY NOTES

DAILY WRAP-UP

NUTRITION NOTES

BY THE NUMBERS **153.9:** Record number of miles run on a treadmill in 24 hours — for a man or woman — set by a Hungarian woman, Edit Berces. **40:** Berces's age when she set the record, in 2004. **7:** Number of miles she ran in the first hour. **3.6:** Miles she ran the final hour.

THURSDAY

MORNING INFO ☐ DAILY RATING ☐

CARDIO EXERCISE	TIME/DISTANCE/INTENSITY	NOTES
_____	_____	_____
_____	_____	_____
_____	_____	_____

STRENGTH TRAINING	WT.	SETS	REPS	NOTES
_____				_____
_____				_____
_____				_____
_____				_____
_____				_____
_____				_____
_____				_____
_____				_____
_____				_____

MIND-BODY NOTES

DAILY WRAP-UP

NUTRITION NOTES

RESEARCH REPORT For treating depression, aerobic exercise and strength training may be as effective as drugs and psychotherapy. In one study, depressed exercisers experienced significantly lower relapse rates than groups who had taken medication.

FRIDAY

MORNING INFO ☐   DAILY RATING ☐

CARDIO EXERCISE	TIME/DISTANCE/INTENSITY	NOTES

STRENGTH TRAINING	WT.	SETS	REPS	NOTES

MIND-BODY NOTES

DAILY WRAP-UP

NUTRITION NOTES

QUICK QUIZ What percentage of Americans eat breakfast? A) 92 percent B) 85 percent C) 74 percent D) 68 percent (Answer on page 212.)

SATURDAY

MORNING INFO

DAILY RATING

CARDIO EXERCISE	TIME/DISTANCE/INTENSITY	NOTES

STRENGTH TRAINING	WT.	SETS	REPS	NOTES

MIND-BODY NOTES

DAILY WRAP-UP

NUTRITION NOTES

TRAINING TRIVIA Hawaii's Ironman triathlon started in 1978 as the result of a bet. Over beers, a group of guys wondered what would happen if they combined the 2.4-mile Waikiki Rough Water Swim, the 112-mile Oahu Bicycle Race, and the Honolulu Marathon.

SUNDAY

MORNING INFO

DAILY RATING

CARDIO EXERCISE	TIME/DISTANCE/INTENSITY	NOTES

STRENGTH TRAINING	WT.	SETS	REPS	NOTES

MIND-BODY NOTES

DAILY WRAP-UP

NUTRITION NOTES

> "The more time you spend doing the things you can do, the less time you have to think about what you can't do." **— MICHEL BOND**, national champion handcyclist

WEEKLY WRAP-UP

WEEKLY
RATING [ ]

Goals: MET _____ EXCEEDED _____ MAYBE NEXT WEEK _____

HIGHLIGHT OF THE WEEK _____

CARDIO NOTES
TOTAL SESSIONS [ ]
MILES/ YARDS [ ]
TOTAL HOURS [ ]

_____

_____

_____

_____

_____

STRENGTH NOTES
TOTAL SESSIONS [ ]

_____

_____

_____

_____

MIND-BODY NOTES

THOUGHTS ABOUT THE WEEK

NUTRITION NOTES _____

_____

_____

_____

WEEK 12

Goals: _____
_____
_____

Dates: _____

MONDAY

MORNING INFO [   ]   DAILY RATING [   ]

CARDIO EXERCISE	TIME/DISTANCE/INTENSITY	NOTES
_____	_____	_____
_____	_____	_____
_____	_____	_____

STRENGTH TRAINING	WT.	SETS	REPS	NOTES
_____				_____
_____				_____
_____				_____
_____				_____
_____				_____
_____				_____
_____				_____
_____				_____
_____				_____
_____				_____

MIND-BODY NOTES

DAILY WRAP-UP

NUTRITION NOTES
_____
_____
_____
_____

MYTH BUSTER Myth: The crunch is the ultimate abdominal exercise. Reality: A crunch performed on a physioball is better: You'll engage more muscle fibers because you have to tense your entire midsection to keep from rolling off the ball.

TUESDAY

MORNING
INFO

DAILY
RATING

CARDIO EXERCISE	TIME/DISTANCE/INTENSITY	NOTES

STRENGTH TRAINING	WT.	SETS	REPS	NOTES

MIND-BODY NOTES

DAILY WRAP-UP

NUTRITION NOTES

NUTRITION NUGGET Residents of the Greek island of Crete circa 1960 got 40 percent of their calories from fat, yet their heart-disease rates were among the world's lowest, largely because the fat they consumed was primarily unsaturated, from olive oil and fish.

WEDNESDAY

MORNING
INFO

DAILY
RATING

CARDIO EXERCISE	TIME/DISTANCE/INTENSITY	NOTES

STRENGTH TRAINING	WT.	SETS	REPS	NOTES

MIND-BODY NOTES

DAILY WRAP-UP

NUTRITION NOTES

BY THE NUMBERS **1900:** First year that women were allowed to compete in the Olympic Games. **1984:** First year that women could run the Olympic marathon. **2000:** First year that women competed in Olympic weightlifting and pole vaulting.

THURSDAY

MORNING INFO

DAILY RATING

CARDIO EXERCISE	TIME/DISTANCE/INTENSITY	NOTES

STRENGTH TRAINING	WT.	SETS	REPS	NOTES

MIND-BODY NOTES

DAILY WRAP-UP

NUTRITION NOTES

RESEARCH REPORT Aerobic exercise increases total sleep time on average by ten minutes per night, according to studies of brain-wave patterns, but it has almost no effect on how quickly people fall asleep or how soundly they sleep.

FRIDAY

MORNING INFO

DAILY RATING

CARDIO EXERCISE	TIME/DISTANCE/INTENSITY	NOTES

STRENGTH TRAINING	WT.	SETS	REPS	NOTES

MIND-BODY NOTES

DAILY WRAP-UP

NUTRITION NOTES

SATURDAY

MORNING INFO

DAILY RATING

CARDIO EXERCISE	TIME/DISTANCE/INTENSITY	NOTES

STRENGTH TRAINING	WT.	SETS	REPS	NOTES

MIND-BODY NOTES

DAILY WRAP-UP

NUTRITION NOTES

TRAINING TRIVIA In the 1800s, treadmills were used as a way of generating power for prisons and as a form of punishment for inmates. Forced to walk up to 12 hours a day, some Australian convicts said they'd rather hang than work their treadmill.

SUNDAY

MORNING INFO [ ] DAILY RATING [ ]

CARDIO EXERCISE	TIME/DISTANCE/INTENSITY	NOTES
_____	_____	_____
_____	_____	_____
_____	_____	_____

STRENGTH TRAINING	WT.	SETS	REPS	NOTES
_____				_____
_____				_____
_____				_____
_____				_____
_____				_____
_____				_____
_____				_____
_____				_____
_____				_____
_____				_____

MIND-BODY NOTES

DAILY WRAP-UP

NUTRITION NOTES

"With my log, I pay more attention to tracking the intangible elements, like my energy and motivation, than the actual workout specifics."
— **MICHELLIE JONES**, 2000 Olympic silver medalist, triathlon

WEEKLY WRAP-UP

WEEKLY RATING ☐

Goals: MET _____ EXCEEDED _____ MAYBE NEXT WEEK _____

HIGHLIGHT OF THE WEEK _____

CARDIO NOTES   TOTAL SESSIONS ☐   MILES/ YARDS ☐   TOTAL HOURS ☐

_____
_____
_____
_____
_____

STRENGTH NOTES   TOTAL SESSIONS ☐

_____
_____
_____
_____

MIND-BODY NOTES	THOUGHTS ABOUT THE WEEK

NUTRITION NOTES _____
_____
_____
_____
_____

WEEK 13

Goals:

Dates:

MONDAY

MORNING INFO

DAILY RATING

CARDIO EXERCISE	TIME/DISTANCE/INTENSITY	NOTES

STRENGTH TRAINING	WT.	SETS	REPS	NOTES

MIND-BODY NOTES

DAILY WRAP-UP

NUTRITION NOTES

MYTH BUSTER **Myth:** Stretching has been proven to prevent injury. **Reality:** Though there are many important reasons to stretch, including maintaining mobility as you age, no scientific evidence has linked stretching to injury prevention.

TUESDAY

MORNING INFO ☐ DAILY RATING ☐

CARDIO EXERCISE	TIME/DISTANCE/INTENSITY	NOTES

STRENGTH TRAINING	WT.	SETS	REPS	NOTES

MIND-BODY NOTES

DAILY WRAP-UP

NUTRITION NOTES

NUTRITION NUGGET Alcohol not only stimulates appetite but also loosens your inhibitions, so you may be less careful about your food choices. Lowest-calorie choice: light beer. A 12-ounce bottle contains about 100 calories.

WEDNESDAY

MORNING INFO

DAILY RATING

CARDIO EXERCISE	TIME/DISTANCE/INTENSITY	NOTES

STRENGTH TRAINING	WT.	SETS	REPS	NOTES

MIND-BODY NOTES

DAILY WRAP-UP

NUTRITION NOTES

BY THE NUMBERS **1,576:** Number of steps up the Empire State Building. **86:** Number of floors climbed in the annual Empire State Building run. **9 minutes, 53 seconds:** Race record. **33:34:** Time run by an 88-year-old man.

THURSDAY

MORNING INFO ☐   DAILY RATING ☐

CARDIO EXERCISE	TIME/DISTANCE/INTENSITY	NOTES
_____	_____	_____
_____	_____	_____
_____	_____	_____

STRENGTH TRAINING	WT.	SETS	REPS	NOTES
_____				_____
_____				_____
_____				_____
_____				_____
_____				_____
_____				_____
_____				_____
_____				_____
_____				_____
_____				_____

MIND-BODY NOTES

DAILY WRAP-UP

NUTRITION NOTES

_____
_____
_____
_____

RESEARCH REPORT A daily hour of moderate exercise can lower your risk of diabetes by nearly 50 percent, primarily by controlling weight and allowing the body to make better use of its insulin. You needn't work out for an hour straight; accumulating the 60 minutes is fine.

FRIDAY

MORNING INFO [ ]

DAILY RATING [ ]

CARDIO EXERCISE	TIME/DISTANCE/INTENSITY	NOTES
_____	_____	_____
_____	_____	_____
_____	_____	_____

STRENGTH TRAINING	WT.	SETS	REPS	NOTES
_____				_____
_____				_____
_____				_____
_____				_____
_____				_____
_____				_____
_____				_____
_____				_____
_____				_____
_____				_____

MIND-BODY NOTES

DAILY WRAP-UP

NUTRITION NOTES

_____
_____
_____
_____

QUICK QUIZ Which of these alcoholic beverages has the fewest calories? **A)** 5 ounces of white wine **B)** a 5-ounce bloody Mary **C)** an 8-ounce gin and tonic **D)** a 3.5-ounce vodka martini (Answer on page 212.)

SATURDAY

MORNING INFO ☐   DAILY RATING ☐

CARDIO EXERCISE	TIME/DISTANCE/INTENSITY	NOTES

STRENGTH TRAINING	WT.	SETS	REPS	NOTES

MIND-BODY NOTES

DAILY WRAP-UP

NUTRITION NOTES

TRAINING TRIVIA The first elliptical trainer was designed by an engineer whose daughter had injured her knee running. To understand her biomechanics, he filmed her jogging on a treadmill; upon plotting a graph of her stride, he noticed it was shaped like an ellipse.

SUNDAY

MORNING
INFO

DAILY
RATING

CARDIO EXERCISE	TIME/DISTANCE/INTENSITY	NOTES

STRENGTH TRAINING	WT.	SETS	REPS	NOTES

MIND-BODY NOTES

DAILY WRAP-UP

NUTRITION NOTES

"What keeps me inspired to train day in and day out is the fact that I always want to improve. It also helps when you set goals that are tough to obtain, but yet realistic." — **DARA TORRES**, four-time Olympian in swimming, four-time gold medalist

WEEKLY WRAP-UP

WEEKLY RATING [ ]

Goals: MET _____ EXCEEDED _____ MAYBE NEXT WEEK _____

HIGHLIGHT OF THE WEEK _____

CARDIO NOTES   TOTAL SESSIONS [ ]   MILES/ YARDS [ ]   TOTAL HOURS [ ]

_____

_____

_____

_____

_____

STRENGTH NOTES   TOTAL SESSIONS [ ]

_____

_____

_____

_____

MIND-BODY NOTES

THOUGHTS ABOUT THE WEEK

NUTRITION NOTES _____

_____

_____

_____

_____

WEEK 14

Goals:

Dates:

MONDAY

MORNING INFO		DAILY RATING	

CARDIO EXERCISE

CARDIO EXERCISE	TIME/DISTANCE/INTENSITY	NOTES

STRENGTH TRAINING

STRENGTH TRAINING	WT.	SETS	REPS	NOTES

MIND-BODY NOTES

DAILY WRAP-UP

NUTRITION NOTES

MYTH BUSTER **Myth:** Fresh vegetables are more nutritious than frozen. **Reality:** Fresh produce that's been sitting in the market or on your counter for a few days may have lost some nutrients. Frozen foods get processed right away so the nutrients are locked in.

TUESDAY

MORNING INFO

DAILY RATING

CARDIO EXERCISE	TIME/DISTANCE/INTENSITY	NOTES

STRENGTH TRAINING	WT.	SETS	REPS	NOTES

MIND-BODY NOTES

DAILY WRAP-UP

NUTRITION NOTES

NUTRITION NUGGET Many restaurant chains don't insist that their cooks use precise measurements — for the size of a lasagna slice or the amount of guacamole on the tostada — so the calorie counts may differ drastically from the numbers posted online or in brochures.

WEDNESDAY

MORNING INFO

DAILY RATING

CARDIO EXERCISE	TIME/DISTANCE/INTENSITY	NOTES

STRENGTH TRAINING	WT.	SETS	REPS	NOTES

MIND-BODY NOTES

DAILY WRAP-UP

NUTRITION NOTES

BY THE NUMBERS **563:** Calories burned per hour while baling hay for a 155-pound person. **317:** Calories burned during house-cleaning. **281:** Calories burned playing hacky sack. **246:** Calories burned walking at a 3-miles-per-hour pace.

THURSDAY

MORNING INFO

DAILY RATING

CARDIO EXERCISE	TIME/DISTANCE/INTENSITY	NOTES

STRENGTH TRAINING	WT.	SETS	REPS	NOTES

MIND-BODY NOTES

DAILY WRAP-UP

NUTRITION NOTES

RESEARCH REPORT Fit women who exercise throughout and after pregnancy tend to weigh the same five years after giving birth as they did before getting pregnant, whereas nonexercisers tend to end up heavier in the long run than they were before momhood.

FRIDAY

MORNING INFO

DAILY RATING

CARDIO EXERCISE	TIME/DISTANCE/INTENSITY	NOTES

STRENGTH TRAINING	WT.	SETS	REPS	NOTES

MIND-BODY NOTES

DAILY WRAP-UP

NUTRITION NOTES

QUICK QUIZ If you order your 16-ounce caffè latte with nonfat milk instead of whole milk, you will save how many calories? **A)** 140 **B)** 100 **C)** 90 **D)** 75 (Answer on page 212.)

SATURDAY

MORNING INFO

DAILY RATING

CARDIO EXERCISE	TIME/DISTANCE/INTENSITY	NOTES
_____	_____	_____
_____	_____	_____
_____	_____	_____
_____	_____	_____

STRENGTH TRAINING	WT.	SETS	REPS	NOTES
_____				_____
_____				_____
_____				_____
_____				_____
_____				_____
_____				_____
_____				_____
_____				_____

MIND-BODY NOTES

DAILY WRAP-UP

NUTRITION NOTES
_____
_____
_____
_____

TRAINING TRIVIA Doctors of the 1890s warned that competitive cyclists could develop a permanent grimace from trying to maintain balance while pedaling hard. They named the condition "bicycle face."

SUNDAY

MORNING INFO ☐   DAILY RATING ☐

CARDIO EXERCISE	TIME/DISTANCE/INTENSITY	NOTES

STRENGTH TRAINING	WT.	SETS	REPS	NOTES

MIND-BODY NOTES

DAILY WRAP-UP

NUTRITION NOTES

"Satisfaction comes not from the achievement but in how we acted through the process. Medals and trophies simply serve as reminders of the journey." — **GORDO BYRN**, 2002 world champion, Ultraman, a 323-mile, triple Ironman triathlon

WEEKLY WRAP-UP

WEEKLY RATING [　]

Goals: MET _____ EXCEEDED _____ MAYBE NEXT WEEK _____

HIGHLIGHT OF THE WEEK _____

CARDIO NOTES   TOTAL SESSIONS [　]   MILES/ YARDS [　]   TOTAL HOURS [　]

_____

_____

_____

_____

_____

STRENGTH NOTES   TOTAL SESSIONS [　]

_____

_____

_____

_____

MIND-BODY NOTES

THOUGHTS ABOUT THE WEEK

NUTRITION NOTES _____

_____

_____

_____

WEEK 15

Goals: _____
_____
_____

Dates: _____

MONDAY

MORNING INFO [   ]   DAILY RATING [   ]

CARDIO EXERCISE	TIME/DISTANCE/INTENSITY	NOTES
_____	_____	_____
_____	_____	_____
_____	_____	_____

STRENGTH TRAINING	WT.	SETS	REPS	NOTES
_____				_____
_____				_____
_____				_____
_____				_____
_____				_____
_____				_____
_____				_____
_____				_____
_____				_____
_____				_____

MIND-BODY NOTES

DAILY WRAP-UP

NUTRITION NOTES
_____
_____
_____
_____

MYTH BUSTER Myth: Vitamins give you energy. **Reality:** Energy can only come from fat, protein, and carbohydrate. Still, since vitamins help convert food energy into a form your body can use, a deficiency may leave you fatigued.

TUESDAY

MORNING INFO		DAILY RATING	

CARDIO EXERCISE	TIME/DISTANCE/INTENSITY	NOTES

STRENGTH TRAINING	WT.	SETS	REPS	NOTES

MIND-BODY NOTES

DAILY WRAP-UP

NUTRITION NOTES

NUTRITION NUGGET Although 90 minutes of consecutive, high-intensity exercise can depress your immune function, you can prevent this by consuming 60 grams of carbohydrate for every hour of strenuous exercise.

WEDNESDAY

MORNING
INFO

DAILY
RATING

CARDIO EXERCISE	TIME/DISTANCE/INTENSITY	NOTES

STRENGTH TRAINING	WT.	SETS	REPS	NOTES

MIND-BODY NOTES

DAILY WRAP-UP

NUTRITION NOTES

BY THE NUMBERS **639:** Number of muscles in the human body. **206:** Number of bones in adult humans. **350:** Number of bones in a baby's body, many of which fuse together by age 12.

THURSDAY

MORNING INFO ☐   DAILY RATING ☐

CARDIO EXERCISE	TIME/DISTANCE/INTENSITY	NOTES
_____	_____	_____
_____	_____	_____
_____	_____	_____
_____	_____	_____

STRENGTH TRAINING	WT.	SETS	REPS	NOTES
_____				_____
_____				_____
_____				_____
_____				_____
_____				_____
_____				_____
_____				_____
_____				_____
_____				_____

MIND-BODY NOTES

DAILY WRAP-UP

NUTRITION NOTES

RESEARCH REPORT Lifting weights improves balance. In a one-year study, middle-aged women who didn't exercise showed an 8.5 percent decline in balance, whereas those who lifted weights improved their balance by 14 percent.

FRIDAY

MORNING INFO

DAILY RATING

CARDIO EXERCISE	TIME/DISTANCE/INTENSITY	NOTES

STRENGTH TRAINING	WT.	SETS	REPS	NOTES

MIND-BODY NOTES

DAILY WRAP-UP

NUTRITION NOTES

QUICK QUIZ A McDonald's Double Cheeseburger contains 490 calories. Which of the following contains more? **A)** Au Bon Pain Almond Croissant **B)** Starbucks Carrot Cake Bar **C)** McDonald's Crispy Chicken Caesar Salad with dressing **D)** all of the above (Answer on page 212.)

SATURDAY

MORNING
INFO

DAILY
RATING

CARDIO EXERCISE	TIME/DISTANCE/INTENSITY	NOTES

STRENGTH TRAINING	WT.	SETS	REPS	NOTES

MIND-BODY NOTES

DAILY WRAP-UP

NUTRITION NOTES

TRAINING TRIVIA The ancient Mayans played an early form of basketball that required keeping the ball in play using everything but their hands. Another key difference from today's game: The losing team was sacrificed.

SUNDAY

MORNING INFO

DAILY RATING

CARDIO EXERCISE	TIME/DISTANCE/INTENSITY	NOTES

STRENGTH TRAINING	WT.	SETS	REPS	NOTES

MIND-BODY NOTES

DAILY WRAP-UP

NUTRITION NOTES

"As you get older, your body doesn't act the same way it did when you were twenty, but you can still accomplish the same things. You just have to use your head a bit more." **— KRISTINE LILLY**,
U.S. National Soccer Team member, three-time Olympian

WEEKLY WRAP-UP

WEEKLY RATING

Goals: MET _____ EXCEEDED _____ MAYBE NEXT WEEK _____

HIGHLIGHT OF THE WEEK _____

CARDIO NOTES   TOTAL SESSIONS   MILES/YARDS   TOTAL HOURS

_____

_____

_____

_____

_____

STRENGTH NOTES   TOTAL SESSIONS

_____

_____

_____

_____

MIND-BODY NOTES

THOUGHTS ABOUT THE WEEK

NUTRITION NOTES _____

_____

_____

_____

_____

WEEK 16

Goals: _____

Dates: _____

MONDAY

MORNING INFO ☐ DAILY RATING ☐

CARDIO EXERCISE

TIME/DISTANCE/INTENSITY

NOTES

STRENGTH TRAINING	WT.	SETS	REPS	NOTES

MIND-BODY NOTES

DAILY WRAP-UP

NUTRITION NOTES

MYTH BUSTER **Myth:** Exercise during pregnancy increases miscarriage risk. **Reality:** Prenatal workouts are not only safe for mom and baby but also can help relieve aches, shorten labor, and speed postpartum recovery. Of course, don't exercise without your doctor's permission.

TUESDAY

MORNING INFO ☐   DAILY RATING ☐

CARDIO EXERCISE	TIME/DISTANCE/INTENSITY	NOTES

STRENGTH TRAINING	WT.	SETS	REPS	NOTES

MIND-BODY NOTES

DAILY WRAP-UP

NUTRITION NOTES

NUTRITION NUGGET Soy may help protect against heart disease and breast cancer, but some soy products contain just 2 percent of the recommended daily amount of calcium, compared to 20 to 30 percent for dairy products. Choose fortified soy milks and yogurts.

WEDNESDAY

MORNING INFO [ ]   DAILY RATING [ ]

CARDIO EXERCISE	TIME/DISTANCE/INTENSITY	NOTES
_____	_____	_____
_____	_____	_____
_____	_____	_____

STRENGTH TRAINING	WT.	SETS	REPS	NOTES
_____				_____
_____				_____
_____				_____
_____				_____
_____				_____
_____				_____
_____				_____
_____				_____
_____				_____

MIND-BODY NOTES

DAILY WRAP-UP

NUTRITION NOTES

BY THE NUMBERS **300 to 500:** Maximum number of miles you should run or walk in athletic shoes before replacing them. **3 to 6:** Maximum number of months you should wear athletic shoes that you use at least three times a week.

THURSDAY

MORNING INFO

DAILY RATING

CARDIO EXERCISE	TIME/DISTANCE/INTENSITY	NOTES

STRENGTH TRAINING	WT.	SETS	REPS	NOTES

MIND-BODY NOTES

DAILY WRAP-UP

NUTRITION NOTES

RESEARCH REPORT In addition to jogging and weight lifting, vertical jumping for two minutes a day may help prevent osteoporosis by increasing hipbone density. But it's hard on the joints and should be done only by men and premenopausal women who don't have osteoporosis.

FRIDAY

MORNING INFO ☐   DAILY RATING ☐

CARDIO EXERCISE	TIME/DISTANCE/INTENSITY	NOTES
_____	_____	_____
_____	_____	_____
_____	_____	_____

STRENGTH TRAINING	WT.	SETS	REPS	NOTES
_____				_____
_____				_____
_____				_____
_____				_____
_____				_____
_____				_____
_____				_____
_____				_____
_____				_____

MIND-BODY NOTES

DAILY WRAP-UP

NUTRITION NOTES
_____
_____
_____

QUICK QUIZ Which of the following contains the most protein?
A) two eggs **B)** one cup of skim milk **C)** one-half cup of tofu **D)** one-half cup of cooked lentils (Answer on page 212.)

SATURDAY

MORNING INFO ☐   DAILY RATING ☐

CARDIO EXERCISE	TIME/DISTANCE/INTENSITY	NOTES

STRENGTH TRAINING	WT.	SETS	REPS	NOTES

MIND-BODY NOTES

DAILY WRAP-UP

NUTRITION NOTES

TRAINING TRIVIA The standard marathon length was established at the 1908 Olympics. The British royal family requested that the marathon, previously 25 miles long, start at Windsor Castle, which was 26.2 miles from the Olympic stadium.

SUNDAY

MORNING INFO [ ]   DAILY RATING [ ]

CARDIO EXERCISE	TIME/DISTANCE/INTENSITY	NOTES

STRENGTH TRAINING	WT.	SETS	REPS	NOTES

MIND-BODY NOTES

DAILY WRAP-UP

NUTRITION NOTES

"You can't have successes without disappointments. I think we all learn that at some point, which helps us handle life's challenges with a positive attitude." **— TIM DEBOOM**, two-time Hawaii Ironman triathlon champion

WEEKLY WRAP-UP
WEEKLY RATING ☐

Goals: MET _____ EXCEEDED _____ MAYBE NEXT WEEK _____

HIGHLIGHT OF THE WEEK _____

CARDIO NOTES   TOTAL SESSIONS ☐   MILES/ YARDS ☐   TOTAL HOURS ☐

_____
_____
_____
_____
_____

STRENGTH NOTES   TOTAL SESSIONS ☐

_____
_____
_____
_____
_____

MIND-BODY NOTES

THOUGHTS ABOUT THE WEEK

NUTRITION NOTES _____
_____
_____
_____
_____

WEEK 17

Goals:

Dates:

MONDAY

MORNING INFO

DAILY RATING

CARDIO EXERCISE	TIME/DISTANCE/INTENSITY	NOTES

STRENGTH TRAINING	WT.	SETS	REPS	NOTES

MIND-BODY NOTES

DAILY WRAP-UP

NUTRITION NOTES

MYTH BUSTER **Myth:** Long, slow workouts are better for weight loss than shorter, more intense ones. **Reality:** What matters is how many calories you burn. The best strategy for weight loss, fitness, and injury prevention is to vary your pace and distance.

TUESDAY

MORNING INFO

DAILY RATING

CARDIO EXERCISE	TIME/DISTANCE/INTENSITY	NOTES

STRENGTH TRAINING	WT.	SETS	REPS	NOTES

MIND-BODY NOTES

DAILY WRAP-UP

NUTRITION NOTES

NUTRITION NUGGET Some regional food brand labels have vastly underestimated calories, fat, and sugar. The Florida government found 75 percent of diet products tested had false information. For instance, a vanilla éclair claiming 2 fat grams actually contained 17.

WEDNESDAY

MORNING INFO

DAILY RATING

CARDIO EXERCISE	TIME/DISTANCE/INTENSITY	NOTES

STRENGTH TRAINING	WT.	SETS	REPS	NOTES

MIND-BODY NOTES

DAILY WRAP-UP

NUTRITION NOTES

BY THE NUMBERS **70 to 90:** Typical resting heart rate of an inactive person. **42 to 60:** Typical resting heart rate of a fit person. **32 to 34:** Resting heart rate of six-time Tour de France champion Lance Armstrong.

THURSDAY

MORNING INFO ☐   DAILY RATING ☐

CARDIO EXERCISE	TIME/DISTANCE/INTENSITY	NOTES

STRENGTH TRAINING	WT.	SETS	REPS	NOTES

MIND-BODY NOTES

DAILY WRAP-UP

NUTRITION NOTES

RESEARCH REPORT Don't trust weight-loss product ads. Of 300 ads surveyed by the Federal Trade Commission, 40 percent contained at least one claim that was almost certainly false; another 55 percent contained statements likely to be false or lacking substantiation.

FRIDAY

MORNING INFO

DAILY RATING

CARDIO EXERCISE	TIME/DISTANCE/INTENSITY	NOTES

STRENGTH TRAINING	WT.	SETS	REPS	NOTES

MIND-BODY NOTES

DAILY WRAP-UP

NUTRITION NOTES

SATURDAY

| MORNING INFO | | DAILY RATING | |

CARDIO EXERCISE	TIME/DISTANCE/INTENSITY	NOTES

STRENGTH TRAINING	WT.	SETS	REPS	NOTES

MIND-BODY NOTES

DAILY WRAP-UP

NUTRITION NOTES

TRAINING TRIVIA The last Olympic gold medals that were made entirely out of gold were awarded in 1912. Today's gold medals are made from pure silver and plated with at least 6 grams of pure gold.

SUNDAY

MORNING INFO [ ]   DAILY RATING [ ]

CARDIO EXERCISE	TIME/DISTANCE/INTENSITY	NOTES
___	___	___
___	___	___
___	___	___

STRENGTH TRAINING	WT.	SETS	REPS	NOTES
___				___
___				___
___				___
___				___
___				___
___				___
___				___
___				___
___				___

MIND-BODY NOTES

DAILY WRAP-UP

NUTRITION NOTES

"Fun should always be the most important goal. If you're short on motivation, you may be fatigued or overstressed."
— **BRAD KEARNS**, professional triathlete and triathlon coach

WEEKLY WRAP-UP

WEEKLY RATING [ ]

Goals: MET _____ EXCEEDED _____ MAYBE NEXT WEEK _____

HIGHLIGHT OF THE WEEK _____

CARDIO NOTES   TOTAL SESSIONS [ ]   MILES/ YARDS [ ]   TOTAL HOURS [ ]

_____

_____

_____

_____

_____

STRENGTH NOTES   TOTAL SESSIONS [ ]

_____

_____

_____

_____

MIND-BODY NOTES

THOUGHTS ABOUT THE WEEK

NUTRITION NOTES _____

_____

_____

_____

_____

WEEK 18

Goals: _____

Dates: _____

MONDAY

MORNING INFO [   ]   DAILY RATING [   ]

CARDIO EXERCISE	TIME/DISTANCE/INTENSITY	NOTES
_____	_____	_____
_____	_____	_____
_____	_____	_____

STRENGTH TRAINING	WT.	SETS	REPS	NOTES
_____				_____
_____				_____
_____				_____
_____				_____
_____				_____
_____				_____
_____				_____
_____				_____
_____				_____

MIND-BODY NOTES

DAILY WRAP-UP

NUTRITION NOTES

MYTH BUSTER Myth: Calories you eat after 7 P.M. turn to fat. Reality: If you eat more calories than you burn, no matter what the clock says, you'll gain fat. If you eat fewer calories than you burn — even if some are consumed during **Nightline** — you'll slim down.

TUESDAY

MORNING INFO ☐ DAILY RATING ☐

CARDIO EXERCISE	TIME/DISTANCE/INTENSITY	NOTES

STRENGTH TRAINING	WT.	SETS	REPS	NOTES

MIND-BODY NOTES

DAILY WRAP-UP

NUTRITION NOTES

NUTRITION NUGGET Carotenoids, pigments found in colorful fruits and vegetables, may help prevent heart disease and cancer and boost immunity. Rich sources include carrots, sweet potatoes, broccoli, collard greens, mangoes, pineapple, peaches, and oranges.

WEDNESDAY

MORNING
INFO

DAILY
RATING

CARDIO EXERCISE	TIME/DISTANCE/INTENSITY	NOTES

STRENGTH TRAINING	WT.	SETS	REPS	NOTES

MIND-BODY NOTES

DAILY WRAP-UP

NUTRITION NOTES

BY THE NUMBERS **188:** Record number of miles run in 24 hours, the equivalent of seven successive marathons. **41:** Age of Yiannis Kouros, when the Greek athlete set the record in 1997. **17 miles:** Distance between his record and the mileage of the second-best finisher.

THURSDAY

MORNING INFO

DAILY RATING

CARDIO EXERCISE	TIME/DISTANCE/INTENSITY	NOTES

STRENGTH TRAINING	WT.	SETS	REPS	NOTES

MIND-BODY NOTES

DAILY WRAP-UP

NUTRITION NOTES

RESEARCH REPORT Social support can help you stick with exercise. In one study, married couples who exercised together had a 14 percent higher attendance rate at a health club than did married people who worked out alone.

FRIDAY

MORNING INFO

DAILY RATING

CARDIO EXERCISE	TIME/DISTANCE/INTENSITY	NOTES

STRENGTH TRAINING	WT.	SETS	REPS	NOTES

MIND-BODY NOTES

DAILY WRAP-UP

NUTRITION NOTES

QUICK QUIZ Nutrition experts recommend limiting artery-clogging fats to approximately 22 grams per day. The average American consumes about how many combined trans and saturated fat grams daily? **A)** 54 **B)** 45 **C)** 36 **D)** 28 (Answer on page 213.)

SATURDAY

MORNING
INFO

DAILY
RATING

CARDIO EXERCISE	TIME/DISTANCE/INTENSITY	NOTES

STRENGTH TRAINING	WT.	SETS	REPS	NOTES

MIND-BODY NOTES

DAILY WRAP-UP

NUTRITION NOTES

TRAINING TRIVIA Golf originated from a fifteenth-century Scottish game that involved hitting a pebble around a course of sand dunes. The term "caddy" was coined in 1552 when avid golfer Mary Queen of Scots called her assistants "cadets."

SUNDAY

MORNING INFO [ ]

DAILY RATING [ ]

CARDIO EXERCISE	TIME/DISTANCE/INTENSITY	NOTES

STRENGTH TRAINING	WT.	SETS	REPS	NOTES

MIND-BODY NOTES

DAILY WRAP-UP

NUTRITION NOTES

"Everyone has days when they don't feel motivated, and usually the anticipation of a workout is always worse than the actual workout, so just get started and it will get better." — **JENNY ADAMS**, champion long jumper and hurdler

WEEKLY WRAP-UP

WEEKLY RATING

Goals: MET _____ EXCEEDED _____ MAYBE NEXT WEEK _____

HIGHLIGHT OF THE WEEK _____

CARDIO NOTES   TOTAL SESSIONS [ ]   MILES/ YARDS [ ]   TOTAL HOURS [ ]

_____

_____

_____

_____

_____

STRENGTH NOTES   TOTAL SESSIONS [ ]

_____

_____

_____

_____

MIND-BODY NOTES

THOUGHTS ABOUT THE WEEK

NUTRITION NOTES _____

_____

_____

_____

WEEK 19

Goals:

Dates:

MONDAY

MORNING INFO

DAILY RATING

CARDIO EXERCISE	TIME/DISTANCE/INTENSITY	NOTES

STRENGTH TRAINING	WT.	SETS	REPS	NOTES

MIND-BODY NOTES

DAILY WRAP-UP

NUTRITION NOTES

MYTH BUSTER **Myth:** Bottom-heavy women should avoid the stairclimber and step aerobics. **Truth:** These are great activities for developing fitness and burning calories, no matter what your body shape. They can help tone your butt without making it larger.

TUESDAY

MORNING INFO

DAILY RATING

CARDIO EXERCISE	TIME/DISTANCE/INTENSITY	NOTES

STRENGTH TRAINING	WT.	SETS	REPS	NOTES

MIND-BODY NOTES

DAILY WRAP-UP

NUTRITION NOTES

NUTRITION NUGGET The two most important nutrients for bone strength are calcium and vitamin D, but eating fruits and vegetables may also help preserve bone-mineral density, perhaps by helping to maintain a good balance of acid in the blood.

WEDNESDAY

MORNING INFO ☐   DAILY RATING ☐

CARDIO EXERCISE	TIME/DISTANCE/INTENSITY	NOTES

STRENGTH TRAINING	WT.	SETS	REPS	NOTES

MIND-BODY NOTES

DAILY WRAP-UP

NUTRITION NOTES

BY THE NUMBERS 12 out of 13: Number of Boston Marathon champions who were Kenyans from 1991 to 2003. 91 out of 100: Number of history's best times in the steeplechase that are held by Kenyans.

THURSDAY

MORNING INFO ☐

DAILY RATING ☐

CARDIO EXERCISE	TIME/DISTANCE/INTENSITY	NOTES
_____	_____	_____
_____	_____	_____
_____	_____	_____

STRENGTH TRAINING	WT.	SETS	REPS	NOTES
_____				_____
_____				_____
_____				_____
_____				_____
_____				_____
_____				_____
_____				_____
_____				_____
_____				_____
_____				

MIND-BODY NOTES

DAILY WRAP-UP

NUTRITION NOTES

RESEARCH REPORT Treadmill running up to 9 miles per hour (a 6:40 pace) burns as many calories as outdoor running. Above 9 mph, treadmill running burns 8 percent fewer calories; you don't have to overcome wind resistance, and the belt propels you a bit.

FRIDAY

MORNING INFO

DAILY RATING

CARDIO EXERCISE	TIME/DISTANCE/INTENSITY	NOTES

STRENGTH TRAINING	WT.	SETS	REPS	NOTES

MIND-BODY NOTES

DAILY WRAP-UP

NUTRITION NOTES

QUICK QUIZ Which has the least trans fat? **A)** half a Marie Callendar's Chicken Pot Pie **B)** six Gorton's Crunchy Golden Fish Sticks **C)** Pillsbury Buttermilk Waffle **D)** Entenmann's Rich Frosted Donut (Answer on page 213.)

SATURDAY

MORNING INFO [ ]

DAILY RATING [ ]

CARDIO EXERCISE	TIME/DISTANCE/INTENSITY	NOTES

STRENGTH TRAINING	WT.	SETS	REPS	NOTES

MIND-BODY NOTES

DAILY WRAP-UP

NUTRITION NOTES

TRAINING TRIVIA The original goal of pole vaulting, formerly called "running pole leaping," was distance rather than height. The ancient Celts used poles to vault over bulls. Europeans used poles to cross canals filled with water.

SUNDAY

MORNING INFO

DAILY RATING

CARDIO EXERCISE	TIME/DISTANCE/INTENSITY	NOTES
_____	_____	_____
_____	_____	_____
_____	_____	_____
_____	_____	_____

STRENGTH TRAINING	WT.	SETS	REPS	NOTES
_____				_____
_____				_____
_____				_____
_____				_____
_____				_____
_____				_____
_____				_____
_____				_____
_____				_____
_____				_____

MIND-BODY NOTES

DAILY WRAP-UP

NUTRITION NOTES

"The first couple trillion times trying to go over the bar were pretty frightening for me." — **STACY DRAGILA**, 2000 Olympic gold medalist, pole vault; world-record holder, women's pole vault

WEEKLY WRAP-UP

WEEKLY RATING ☐

Goals: MET _____ EXCEEDED _____ MAYBE NEXT WEEK _____

HIGHLIGHT OF THE WEEK _____

CARDIO NOTES   TOTAL SESSIONS ☐   MILES/ YARDS ☐   TOTAL HOURS ☐

_____
_____
_____
_____
_____

STRENGTH NOTES   TOTAL SESSIONS ☐

_____
_____
_____
_____

MIND-BODY NOTES

THOUGHTS ABOUT THE WEEK

NUTRITION NOTES _____
_____
_____
_____

WEEK 20

Goals: _____
_____
_____
_____

Dates: _____

MONDAY

MORNING INFO [ ]   DAILY RATING [ ]

CARDIO EXERCISE	TIME/DISTANCE/INTENSITY	NOTES
_____	_____	_____
_____	_____	_____
_____	_____	_____

STRENGTH TRAINING	WT.	SETS	REPS	NOTES
_____				_____
_____				_____
_____				_____
_____				_____
_____				_____
_____				_____
_____				_____
_____				_____
_____				_____
_____				_____

MIND-BODY NOTES

DAILY WRAP-UP

NUTRITION NOTES
_____
_____
_____
_____

MYTH BUSTER **Myth:** You should lose weight before lifting weights. **Reality:** Strength training may help you slim down, since it will help preserve (or even increase) your metabolism. Plus, with stronger muscles, you'll have more oomph for cardio activities.

TUESDAY

MORNING INFO [ ]   DAILY RATING [ ]

CARDIO EXERCISE	TIME/DISTANCE/INTENSITY	NOTES
_____	_____	_____
_____	_____	_____
_____	_____	_____

STRENGTH TRAINING	WT.	SETS	REPS	NOTES
_____				_____
_____				_____
_____				_____
_____				_____
_____				_____
_____				_____
_____				_____
_____				_____
_____				_____

MIND-BODY NOTES

DAILY WRAP-UP

NUTRITION NOTES
_____
_____
_____
_____

NUTRITION NUGGET The terms "enriched" and "fortified" aren't synonymous. **Enriched** means that nutrients lost during processing have been added back in. **Fortified** indicates that nutrients not originally present have been added, such as vitamin D in milk.

WEDNESDAY

MORNING INFO

DAILY RATING

CARDIO EXERCISE	TIME/DISTANCE/INTENSITY	NOTES

STRENGTH TRAINING	WT.	SETS	REPS	NOTES

MIND-BODY NOTES

DAILY WRAP-UP

NUTRITION NOTES

BY THE NUMBERS 18,425: Average number of steps per day (about 9 miles) walked by Amish men. 14,196: Number of daily steps walked by Amish women (about 7 miles). 0: Percentage of Amish men considered obese. 9: Percentage of Amish women considered obese.

THURSDAY

MORNING INFO ☐   DAILY RATING ☐

CARDIO EXERCISE	TIME/DISTANCE/INTENSITY	NOTES

STRENGTH TRAINING	WT.	SETS	REPS	NOTES

MIND-BODY NOTES

DAILY WRAP-UP

NUTRITION NOTES

RESEARCH REPORT Compared to men who watch TV an hour or less per week, men who tuned in for 2 to 10 hours per week had a 66 percent greater risk for diabetes. Men who watched 21 to 40 hours had double the risk.

FRIDAY

MORNING INFO ____

DAILY RATING ____

CARDIO EXERCISE	TIME/DISTANCE/INTENSITY	NOTES

STRENGTH TRAINING	WT.	SETS	REPS	NOTES

MIND-BODY NOTES

DAILY WRAP-UP

NUTRITION NOTES

QUICK QUIZ Which has the fewest calories? **A)** four pancakes plus one-fourth cup syrup **B)** Belgian waffle with fruit and whipped topping **C)** three French toast slices with one-fourth cup syrup **D)** ham and cheese omelet with three eggs (Answer on page 213.)

SATURDAY

MORNING INFO ☐   DAILY RATING ☐

CARDIO EXERCISE	TIME/DISTANCE/INTENSITY	NOTES

STRENGTH TRAINING	WT.	SETS	REPS	NOTES

MIND-BODY NOTES

DAILY WRAP-UP

NUTRITION NOTES

TRAINING TRIVIA The earliest organized soccer games featured goals as many as four miles apart. By 1801, the playing area had been confined to between 80 and 100 yards, with a goal at each end made of two sticks and tape stretched between them.

SUNDAY

MORNING INFO [ ]   DAILY RATING [ ]

CARDIO EXERCISE	TIME/DISTANCE/INTENSITY	NOTES

STRENGTH TRAINING	WT.	SETS	REPS	NOTES

MIND-BODY NOTES

DAILY WRAP-UP

NUTRITION NOTES

"I feel it is important to actually write your goals on paper. This process makes your expectations become more tangible and realistic. I usually read over them about once a month or before a competition."
— **ALAN CULPEPPER**, 2004 Olympic marathoner

WEEKLY WRAP-UP

WEEKLY RATING ☐

Goals: MET _____ EXCEEDED _____ MAYBE NEXT WEEK _____

HIGHLIGHT OF THE WEEK _____

CARDIO NOTES   TOTAL SESSIONS ☐   MILES/ YARDS ☐   TOTAL HOURS ☐

_____

_____

_____

_____

_____

STRENGTH NOTES   TOTAL SESSIONS ☐

_____

_____

_____

_____

MIND-BODY NOTES

THOUGHTS ABOUT THE WEEK

NUTRITION NOTES _____

_____

_____

_____

_____

WEEK 21

Goals:

Dates:

MONDAY

MORNING INFO

DAILY RATING

CARDIO EXERCISE	TIME/DISTANCE/INTENSITY	NOTES

STRENGTH TRAINING	WT.	SETS	REPS	NOTES

MIND-BODY NOTES

DAILY WRAP-UP

NUTRITION NOTES

MYTH BUSTER **Myth:** Beginning weightlifters should stick to machines. **Reality:** Most free-weight exercises are quite safe for novices. Plus, they work many deeper muscles not challenged by machines and help to develop balance and coordination.

TUESDAY

MORNING INFO ☐   DAILY RATING ☐

CARDIO EXERCISE	TIME/DISTANCE/INTENSITY	NOTES
_____	_____	_____
_____	_____	_____
_____	_____	_____

STRENGTH TRAINING	WT.	SETS	REPS	NOTES
_____				_____
_____				_____
_____				_____
_____				_____
_____				_____
_____				_____
_____				_____
_____				_____
_____				_____

MIND-BODY NOTES

DAILY WRAP-UP

NUTRITION NOTES

_____
_____
_____
_____

NUTRITION NUGGET On a typical diet, the maximum number of combined saturated and trans fat grams recommended per day is 22. A Burger King Whopper with cheese alone has 29 grams of artery-clogging fat.

WEDNESDAY

MORNING INFO ☐   DAILY RATING ☐

CARDIO EXERCISE	TIME/DISTANCE/INTENSITY	NOTES
_____	_____	_____
_____	_____	_____
_____	_____	_____

STRENGTH TRAINING	WT.	SETS	REPS	NOTES
_____				_____
_____				_____
_____				_____
_____				_____
_____				_____
_____				_____
_____				_____
_____				_____
_____				_____

MIND-BODY NOTES

DAILY WRAP-UP

NUTRITION NOTES

_____

_____

_____

_____

THURSDAY

MORNING INFO

DAILY RATING

CARDIO EXERCISE	TIME/DISTANCE/INTENSITY	NOTES

STRENGTH TRAINING	WT.	SETS	REPS	NOTES

MIND-BODY NOTES

DAILY WRAP-UP

NUTRITION NOTES

RESEARCH REPORT Fit women who exercise through pregnancy tend to have shorter labors than sedentary women, although there are no guarantees. In one study, 65 percent of exercisers delivered in less than four hours, compared to 31 percent of nonexercisers.

FRIDAY

MORNING INFO [ ]   DAILY RATING [ ]

CARDIO EXERCISE	TIME/DISTANCE/INTENSITY	NOTES
_____	_____	_____
_____	_____	_____
_____	_____	_____

STRENGTH TRAINING	WT.	SETS	REPS	NOTES
_____				_____
_____				_____
_____				_____
_____				_____
_____				_____
_____				_____
_____				_____
_____				_____
_____				_____

MIND-BODY NOTES

DAILY WRAP-UP

NUTRITION NOTES
_____
_____
_____
_____

QUICK QUIZ Which vegetable, when boiled, has the most fiber per half cup? **A)** broccoli **B)** asparagus **C)** spinach **D)** Brussels sprouts (Answer on page 213.)

SATURDAY

MORNING
INFO

DAILY
RATING

CARDIO EXERCISE	TIME/DISTANCE/INTENSITY	NOTES

STRENGTH TRAINING	WT.	SETS	REPS	NOTES

MIND-BODY NOTES

DAILY WRAP-UP

NUTRITION NOTES

TRAINING TRIVIA Drawings of swimmers doing the breast-stroke — or, perhaps, the dog paddle — dating from the Stone Age have been found in Egyptian caves. Records suggest the first swimming competitions were held in 36 B.C.E., organized by a Japanese emperor.

SUNDAY

MORNING
INFO

DAILY
RATING

CARDIO EXERCISE	TIME/DISTANCE/INTENSITY	NOTES
_____	_____	_____
_____	_____	_____
_____	_____	_____

STRENGTH TRAINING	WT.	SETS	REPS	NOTES
_____				_____
_____				_____
_____				_____
_____				_____
_____				_____
_____				_____
_____				_____
_____				_____
_____				_____
_____				

MIND-BODY NOTES

DAILY WRAP-UP

NUTRITION NOTES

_____

_____

_____

_____

"Whatever sport or activity you do, you have to do it for yourself — not your parents or your friends or anyone else." — **MEGAN QUANN**, two-time Olympic gold medalist, breaststroke

WEEKLY WRAP-UP

WEEKLY RATING

Goals: MET _____ EXCEEDED _____ MAYBE NEXT WEEK _____

HIGHLIGHT OF THE WEEK _____

CARDIO NOTES   TOTAL SESSIONS ☐   MILES/ YARDS ☐   TOTAL HOURS ☐

_____

_____

_____

_____

_____

STRENGTH NOTES   TOTAL SESSIONS ☐

_____

_____

_____

_____

MIND-BODY NOTES

THOUGHTS ABOUT THE WEEK

NUTRITION NOTES _____

_____

_____

_____

WEEK 22

Goals:

Dates:

MONDAY

| MORNING INFO | | DAILY RATING | |

CARDIO EXERCISE	TIME/DISTANCE/INTENSITY	NOTES

STRENGTH TRAINING	WT.	SETS	REPS	NOTES

MIND-BODY NOTES

DAILY WRAP-UP

NUTRITION NOTES

MYTH BUSTER **Myth:** The longer you hold a stretch, the more flexible you'll become. **Reality:** Stretching for 30 seconds seems to improve flexibility just as well as stretching for 60 seconds, although 30 seconds does seem to be more effective than 15.

TUESDAY

MORNING INFO

DAILY RATING

CARDIO EXERCISE	TIME/DISTANCE/INTENSITY	NOTES

STRENGTH TRAINING	WT.	SETS	REPS	NOTES

MIND-BODY NOTES

DAILY WRAP-UP

NUTRITION NOTES

NUTRITION NUGGET Vegetarians have many nutritious high-protein options, including beans (15 grams per cup), tofu (10 grams), and hummus (6 grams per half cup). Veggie burgers and meatless breakfast patties made of soy protein generally have 7 to 14 grams of protein each.

WEDNESDAY

MORNING INFO ☐   DAILY RATING ☐

CARDIO EXERCISE	TIME/DISTANCE/INTENSITY	NOTES

STRENGTH TRAINING	WT.	SETS	REPS	NOTES

MIND-BODY NOTES

DAILY WRAP-UP

NUTRITION NOTES

BY THE NUMBERS 28 mph: Typical swimming speed of salmon. 5.2 mph: Speed of top male swimmers in the 50-meter freestyle. 5 mph: Swimming speed of cod. 4.6 mph: Speed of top female swimmers. 3.7 mph: Speed of herring.

THURSDAY

MORNING INFO

DAILY RATING

CARDIO EXERCISE	TIME/DISTANCE/INTENSITY	NOTES

STRENGTH TRAINING	WT.	SETS	REPS	NOTES

MIND-BODY NOTES

DAILY WRAP-UP

NUTRITION NOTES

RESEARCH REPORT Overweight men and those who ride more than ten hours a week are at greater risk for experiencing cycling-related impotence, but specially designed seats may help solve the problem.

FRIDAY

MORNING INFO

DAILY RATING

CARDIO EXERCISE	TIME/DISTANCE/INTENSITY	NOTES

STRENGTH TRAINING	WT.	SETS	REPS	NOTES

MIND-BODY NOTES

DAILY WRAP-UP

NUTRITION NOTES

QUICK QUIZ One large egg contains 75 calories and 5 grams of fat. How much of that fat is of the artery-clogging, saturated variety? **A)** 5 grams **B)** 4.2 grams **C)** 3.2 grams **D)** 1.6 grams (Answer on page 213.)

SATURDAY

MORNING INFO ☐   DAILY RATING ☐

CARDIO EXERCISE	TIME/DISTANCE/INTENSITY	NOTES
_____	_____	_____
_____	_____	_____
_____	_____	_____
_____		

STRENGTH TRAINING	WT.	SETS	REPS	NOTES
_____				_____
_____				_____
_____				_____
_____				_____
_____				_____
_____				_____
_____				_____
_____				_____

MIND-BODY NOTES

DAILY WRAP-UP

NUTRITION NOTES

TRAINING TRIVIA The first archaeological evidence of yoga's existence is found in stone artifacts depicting figures performing yoga postures. These artifacts, excavated from a valley in India, appear to date from 3000 B.C.E.

SUNDAY

MORNING INFO ☐   DAILY RATING ☐

CARDIO EXERCISE	TIME/DISTANCE/INTENSITY	NOTES
_____	_____	_____
_____	_____	_____
_____	_____	_____

STRENGTH TRAINING	WT.	SETS	REPS	NOTES
_____				_____
_____				_____
_____				_____
_____				_____
_____				_____
_____				_____
_____				_____
_____				_____
_____				_____
_____				_____

MIND-BODY NOTES

DAILY WRAP-UP

NUTRITION NOTES

"I always write my goals down. It makes them seem like something I expect to accomplish rather than just something I hope happens."
— **DAVID BAILEY**, 2000 Hawaii Ironman triathlon champion, handcycle division

WEEKLY WRAP-UP

WEEKLY RATING [ ]

Goals: MET _____ EXCEEDED _____ MAYBE NEXT WEEK _____

HIGHLIGHT OF THE WEEK _____

CARDIO NOTES   TOTAL SESSIONS [ ]   MILES/ YARDS [ ]   TOTAL HOURS [ ]

_____

_____

_____

_____

_____

STRENGTH NOTES   TOTAL SESSIONS [ ]

_____

_____

_____

_____

MIND-BODY NOTES

THOUGHTS ABOUT THE WEEK

NUTRITION NOTES _____

_____

_____

_____

WEEK 23

Goals: _____

Dates: _____

MONDAY

MORNING INFO ☐   DAILY RATING ☐

CARDIO EXERCISE	TIME/DISTANCE/INTENSITY	NOTES

STRENGTH TRAINING	WT.	SETS	REPS	NOTES

MIND-BODY NOTES

DAILY WRAP-UP

NUTRITION NOTES

MYTH BUSTER **Myth:** You can reduce your love handles by twisting from side to side. **Reality:** Side twists don't reduce fat and are risky for your lower back. They're not even an effective way to strengthen your obliques, the muscles that wrap around your sides.

TUESDAY

MORNING INFO

DAILY RATING

CARDIO EXERCISE	TIME/DISTANCE/INTENSITY	NOTES

STRENGTH TRAINING	WT.	SETS	REPS	NOTES

MIND-BODY NOTES

DAILY WRAP-UP

NUTRITION NOTES

NUTRITION NUGGET Don't assume a bread labeled "wheat" or "12 grain" is high in fiber. It might be 90 percent white flour with caramel coloring and a few sprinkles of whole grain. Look for at least 3 grams of fiber per slice.

WEDNESDAY

MORNING INFO

DAILY RATING

CARDIO EXERCISE	TIME/DISTANCE/INTENSITY	NOTES
_____	_____	_____
_____	_____	_____
_____	_____	_____

STRENGTH TRAINING	WT.	SETS	REPS	NOTES
_____				_____
_____				_____
_____				_____
_____				_____
_____				_____
_____				_____
_____				_____
_____				_____
_____				_____

MIND-BODY NOTES

DAILY WRAP-UP

NUTRITION NOTES

_____

_____

_____

_____

_____

BY THE NUMBERS **11:** Percentage of body fat of cyclists starting the 2,910-mile Race Across America. **4:** Percentage of body fat after completing RAAM, in an average time of 239 hours. **176:** Average level of total cholesterol at the race start. **133:** Finishing total cholesterol.

THURSDAY

MORNING INFO ☐   DAILY RATING ☐

CARDIO EXERCISE	TIME/DISTANCE/INTENSITY	NOTES
_____	_____	_____
_____	_____	_____
_____	_____	_____
_____		_____

STRENGTH TRAINING	WT.	SETS	REPS	NOTES
_____				_____
_____				_____
_____				_____
_____				_____
_____				_____
_____				_____
_____				_____
_____				_____
_____				_____

MIND-BODY NOTES

DAILY WRAP-UP

NUTRITION NOTES

RESEARCH REPORT Exercise is good for your brain. Adults who walked three times a week for up to 45 minutes saw an 11 percent improvement on tests measuring decision-making ability. Other studies show improved memory among exercisers.

FRIDAY

MORNING INFO

DAILY RATING

CARDIO EXERCISE	TIME/DISTANCE/INTENSITY	NOTES

STRENGTH TRAINING	WT.	SETS	REPS	NOTES

MIND-BODY NOTES

DAILY WRAP-UP

NUTRITION NOTES

QUICK QUIZ Which of the following Panda Express dishes, in 5-ounce servings, contain less than 350 calories? **A)** chicken with mushrooms **B)** beef and broccoli **C)** orange chicken **D)** all of the above (Answer on page 213.)

SATURDAY

MORNING INFO ☐   DAILY RATING ☐

CARDIO EXERCISE	TIME/DISTANCE/INTENSITY	NOTES
_____	_____	_____
_____	_____	_____
_____	_____	_____

STRENGTH TRAINING	WT.	SETS	REPS	NOTES
_____				_____
_____				_____
_____				_____
_____				_____
_____				_____
_____				_____
_____				_____
_____				_____
_____				_____

MIND-BODY NOTES

DAILY WRAP-UP

NUTRITION NOTES

TRAINING TRIVIA Gymnastics has been around for more than 2,000 years, but as a competitive sport it is barely a century old. Early competitions included the pole vault and broad jump, but by the 1950s, track and field events had disappeared from gymnastic competitions.

SUNDAY

MORNING INFO

DAILY RATING

CARDIO EXERCISE	TIME/DISTANCE/INTENSITY	NOTES

STRENGTH TRAINING	WT.	SETS	REPS	NOTES

MIND-BODY NOTES

DAILY WRAP-UP

NUTRITION NOTES

"I love being out in the sunshine, I love being with my teammates, and I love to be around the soccer ball, which makes it very easy to motivate myself." **— LANDON DONOVAN**, member 2000 Olympic soccer team, 2002 World Cup All-Star team

WEEKLY WRAP-UP

WEEKLY RATING ☐

Goals: MET _____ EXCEEDED _____ MAYBE NEXT WEEK _____

HIGHLIGHT OF THE WEEK _____

CARDIO NOTES   TOTAL SESSIONS ☐   MILES/ YARDS ☐   TOTAL HOURS ☐

_____

_____

_____

_____

_____

STRENGTH NOTES   TOTAL SESSIONS ☐

_____

_____

_____

_____

MIND-BODY NOTES

THOUGHTS ABOUT THE WEEK

NUTRITION NOTES _____

_____

_____

_____

_____

WEEK 24

Goals: _____

_____

_____

Dates: _____

MONDAY

MORNING INFO [ ]   **DAILY RATING** [ ]

CARDIO EXERCISE	TIME/DISTANCE/INTENSITY	NOTES
_____	_____	_____
_____	_____	_____
_____	_____	_____

STRENGTH TRAINING	WT.	SETS	REPS	NOTES
_____				_____
_____				_____
_____				_____
_____				_____
_____				_____
_____				_____
_____				_____
_____				_____
_____				_____
_____				_____

MIND-BODY NOTES

DAILY WRAP-UP

NUTRITION NOTES

_____

_____

_____

_____

MYTH BUSTER Myth: If you don't feel sore after exercise, you're not getting stronger. **Reality:** Consistent soreness isn't a good sign. It means you haven't recovered from your previous workout. You shouldn't feel sore except after a new or especially tough workout.

TUESDAY

MORNING INFO

DAILY RATING

CARDIO EXERCISE	TIME/DISTANCE/INTENSITY	NOTES

STRENGTH TRAINING	WT.	SETS	REPS	NOTES

MIND-BODY NOTES

DAILY WRAP-UP

NUTRITION NOTES

NUTRITION NUGGET The iron in plant foods isn't well absorbed, so vegetarians may need twice the recommended 15 mg of iron per day. Good plant sources include spinach (3 mg per half cup), beans (3 mg per half cup lentils), and fortified breakfast cereals (2 mg to 10 mg per half cup).

WEDNESDAY

MORNING INFO

DAILY RATING

CARDIO EXERCISE	TIME/DISTANCE/INTENSITY	NOTES

STRENGTH TRAINING	WT.	SETS	REPS	NOTES

MIND-BODY NOTES

DAILY WRAP-UP

NUTRITION NOTES

BY THE NUMBERS **26.2:** Percentage of the U.S. population that gets the recommended amount of exercise — 30 minutes a day on most days of the week. **27:** Percentage of Americans who are totally inactive.

THURSDAY

MORNING INFO ☐ DAILY RATING ☐

CARDIO EXERCISE	TIME/DISTANCE/INTENSITY	NOTES
_____	_____	_____
_____	_____	_____
_____	_____	_____

STRENGTH TRAINING	WT.	SETS	REPS	NOTES
_____				_____
_____				_____
_____				_____
_____				_____
_____				_____
_____				_____
_____				_____
_____				_____
_____				_____

MIND-BODY NOTES

DAILY WRAP-UP

NUTRITION NOTES

RESEARCH REPORT Cardiovascular exercise is especially effective in whittling your middle. Research shows that among men with the same height and weight, the more fit men have less abdominal fat, the type linked with disease risk.

FRIDAY

MORNING
INFO

DAILY
RATING

CARDIO EXERCISE	TIME/DISTANCE/INTENSITY	NOTES
_____	_____	_____
_____	_____	_____
_____	_____	_____
_____	_____	_____

STRENGTH TRAINING	WT.	SETS	REPS	NOTES
_____				_____
_____				_____
_____				_____
_____				_____
_____				_____
_____				_____
_____				_____
_____				_____
_____				_____

MIND-BODY NOTES

DAILY WRAP-UP

NUTRITION NOTES

QUICK QUIZ Which of the following cereals is the only one that contains any fiber? **A)** General Mills Rice Chex **B)** Kellogg's Frosted Flakes **C)** Kellogg's Rice Krispies **D)** General Mills Total Corn Flakes (Answer on page 213.)

SATURDAY

MORNING INFO [   ]   DAILY RATING [   ]

CARDIO EXERCISE	TIME/DISTANCE/INTENSITY	NOTES

STRENGTH TRAINING	WT.	SETS	REPS	NOTES

MIND-BODY NOTES

DAILY WRAP-UP

NUTRITION NOTES

TRAINING TRIVIA Exercise, according to one 1860s educator, would help women produce a "sound nervous system . . . destroying the tendency to mental irritability and hysteria."

SUNDAY

MORNING INFO [ ]   DAILY RATING [ ]

CARDIO EXERCISE	TIME/DISTANCE/INTENSITY	NOTES
_____	_____	_____
_____	_____	_____
_____	_____	_____

STRENGTH TRAINING	WT.	SETS	REPS	NOTES
_____				_____
_____				_____
_____				_____
_____				_____
_____				_____
_____				_____
_____				_____
_____				_____
_____				_____

MIND-BODY NOTES

DAILY WRAP-UP

NUTRITION NOTES

"One lesson I've learned about training is that you only get out of it what you put in." **— MELISSA MORRISON**, 2000 Olympic bronze medalist, 100-meter hurdles

WEEKLY WRAP-UP

WEEKLY RATING ☐

Goals: MET _____ EXCEEDED _____ MAYBE NEXT WEEK _____

HIGHLIGHT OF THE WEEK _____

CARDIO NOTES   TOTAL SESSIONS ☐   MILES/ YARDS ☐   TOTAL HOURS ☐

_____

_____

_____

_____

_____

STRENGTH NOTES   TOTAL SESSIONS ☐

_____

_____

_____

_____

MIND-BODY NOTES

THOUGHTS ABOUT THE WEEK

NUTRITION NOTES _____

_____

_____

_____

_____

Quick Quiz Answers

Here are the answers to the Saturday nutrition quizzes.

WEEK 1
ANSWER: B. The sausage contains 340 calories; the hash browns, 220; the ham, 200; and the bacon, 140.

WEEK 2
ANSWER: A.

WEEK 3
ANSWER: A. The onion contains 1,690 calories and 44 grams of artery-clogging fat (saturated plus trans fat); the wings, 1,010 calories and 22 grams of artery-clogging fat; and the skins, 1,120 calories and 48 grams of artery-clogging fat.

WEEK 4
ANSWER: C. Plain nonfat yogurt has 430 mg of calcium; milk, 300; cottage cheese, 126; spinach, 244.

WEEK 5
ANSWER: D. The shortrib has 20.2 grams of saturated fat; the porterhouse steak, 10.1; the broiled top sirloin, 3.4; the roasted eye of round, 2.3.

WEEK 6
ANSWER: C.

WEEK 7
ANSWER: B.

WEEK 8
ANSWER: A. Milbrook's Cracked Wheat Bread, with 0 grams of fiber per slice. The Oroweat 12 Grain Bread contains 1 gram; the Wonder Bread, 1 gram; and the Pepperidge Farm Very Thin Sliced Wheat Bread, 1.5.

WEEK 9
ANSWER: C. The pear, with 4.3 grams of fiber. The apple contains 3 grams; the cup of blueberries, 3.4; and the banana, 1.8.

WEEK 10
ANSWER: D.

WEEK 11
ANSWER: B.

WEEK 12
ANSWER: C.

WEEK 13
ANSWER: A. A 5-ounce glass of white wine contains 105 to 110 calories; a 5-ounce bloody Mary, 125 calories; an 8-ounce gin and tonic, 155 calories; a 3.5-ounce martini, 140.

WEEK 14
ANSWER: B.

WEEK 15
ANSWER: D. The Au Bon Pain Almond Croissant contains 570 calories; Starbucks Carrot Cake Bar, 540; McDonald's Crispy Chicken Caesar Salad with dressing, 500.

WEEK 16
ANSWER: A. Two eggs contain 12.4 grams of protein; 1 cup of skim milk, 8.3 grams; ½ cup tofu, 9.8 grams; ½ cup cooked lentils, 7.8.

WEEK 17
ANSWER: B.

WEEK 18
ANSWER: D.

WEEK 19
ANSWER: C. Pillsbury Buttermilk Waffle has 1.5 grams of trans fat; half a Marie Callendar's Chicken Pot Pie, 8; six Gorton's Crunchy Golden Fish Sticks, 3; Entenmann's Rich Frosted Donut, 4.

WEEK 20
ANSWER: D. A ham and cheese omelet with three eggs contains 510 calories; a Belgian waffle with fruit and whipped topping contains 900; four pancakes plus ¼ cup syrup, 870; three French toast slices with ¼ cup syrup, 800.

WEEK 21
ANSWER: D. Brussels sprouts contain 3.4 grams of fiber; broccoli, 2 grams; asparagus, .8 grams; spinach, 2 grams.

WEEK 22
ANSWER: D.

WEEK 23
ANSWER: D. At Panda Express, chicken with mushrooms contains 170 calories; beef and broccoli, 180 calories; orange chicken, 310 calories.

WEEK 24
ANSWER: B. The Frosted Flakes contain 1 gram of fiber per serving. All of the others contain none.

How Many Calories Do You Burn?

This chart provides an estimate of the number of calories you'll burn per hour doing different activities. Keep in mind that the numbers vary depending on your weight, metabolism, and muscle mass.

	CALORIES BURNED PER HOUR	
ACTIVITY	135-POUND PERSON	180-POUND PERSON
Aerobic dance		
moderate intensity	329	443
high intensity	549	738
Basketball		
(not counting breaks)	512	689
Bicycling (outdoors)		
12 mph	483	649
15 mph	604	812
18 mph	725	974
Golf (no cart)	293	394
Running		
10-minute miles	589	877
9-minute miles	718	965
8-minute miles	800	1,075
7-minute miles	905	1,216
Rowing	392	526
Swimming		
crawl, 35 yards/minute	396	528
crawl, 50 yards/minute	570	768
breaststroke, 30 yards/minute	384	516
breaststroke, 40 yards/minute	516	690
Tennis		
singles	399	536
doubles	146	197
Walking		
20-minute miles	211	284
15-minute miles	260	350
Circuit weight training (not including rest)	439	590

Workout Ratings:
The Big Picture

At the end of each week, record your daily and weekly ratings here. This chart will help you see weekly and monthly patterns in your training. You might notice, for instance, that you perform better when you rest two days rather than one or when you take one extra-easy week each month. If you get injured, a glance at your chart might help explain why.

WEEK	M	T	W	T	F	S	S	WEEKLY
1								
2								
3								
4								
5								
6								
7								
8								
9								
10								
11								
12								
13								
14								
15								
16								
17								
18								
19								
20								
21								
22								
23								
24								

Personal Records

Don't think that the only place to set a record is in a competition. Use this chart to log breakthroughs in your workouts—whether it's the first time you bench-press 120 pounds, cycle 50 miles, or exercise five times in one week.

DATE	ACTIVITY	ACCOMPLISHMENT

Six-month Wrap-up

Congrats! You've completed your log. Before you start your next diary, take some time to see what you've accomplished over the last six months. Did you meet your goals? Jotting down the answer here will help you set new ones.

➡ **OVERALL GOALS**

➡ **CARDIO EXERCISE GOALS**

➡ **STRENGTH-TRAINING GOALS**

➡ **NUTRITION GOALS**

➡ **MIND-BODY GOALS**

Resources

BOOKS

The following books can expand your knowledge of fitness and your repertoire of exercises.

A Woman's Book of Strength, Karen Andes, Perigee, 1995.

Athletic Abs, Scott Cole and Tom Seabourne, Ph.D., Human Kinetics, 2002.

Core Performance, Mark Verstegen, Rodale Press, 2004.

The Cyclist's Training Bible, Joe Friel, Velo Press, 2003.

The Fat-Free Truth, Liz Neporent, M.A., and Suzanne Schlosberg, Houghton Mifflin Company, 2005.

Fitness for Dummies, Liz Neporent, M.A., and Suzanne Schlosberg, John Wiley & Sons, 2005.

The Heart Rate Guidebook to Heart Zone Training, Sally Edwards, Heart Zone Publishing, 1999.

Instant Stretch, Mark Evans, Barnes & Noble Books, 2001.

Jennifer Kries's Pilates Plus Method, Jennifer Kries, Warner Books, 2002.

The Pilates Body, Brooke Siler, Broadway Books, 2000.

The Pilates Edge, Karrie Adamany and Daniel Loigerot, Penguin Books, 2004.

Slow Fat Triathlete, Jayne Williams, Marlowe & Company, 2004.

The Triathlete's Training Bible, Joe Friel, Velo Press, 2004.

The Ultimate Body, Liz Neporent, Ballantine, 2003.

The Ultimate Body Rolling Workout, Yamuna Zake and Stephanie Golden, Broadway Books, 2004.

Weight Training for Dummies, Liz Neporent and Suzanne Schlosberg, John Wiley & Sons, 2000.

The Wharton's Stretch Book, Jim and Phil Wharton, Times Books, 1996.

Yoga: Mastering the Basics, Sandra Anderson and Rolf Sovik, The Himalayan Institute Press, 2000.

WEB SITES

The following Web sites can help you locate a certified personal trainer or coach, plan a training program on your own, and research various aspects of fitness and nutrition.

Aerobics and Fitness Association of America
www.afaa.com

American College of Sports Medicine
www.acsm.org

American Council on Exercise
www.acefitness.org

American Dietetic Association
www.eatright.org

Center for Science in the Public Interest
www.cspinet.org

Heart Zones Training
www.heartzone.com

National Strength and Conditioning Association
www.nsca-lift.org

Training Bible
www.trainingbible.com

U.S. Department of Agriculture's Nutrient Database for Standard Reference
www.nal.usda.gov/fnic/foodcomp/search/

Yoga Alliance
www.yogaalliance.org

Sources

SETTING YOUR GOALS

Judy L. Van Raalte and Britton W. Brewer (editors), *Exploring Sport and Exercise Psychology,* Chapter 3: "Goal Setting in Sport and Exercise: Research to Practice," pp. 25–48.

Robert Weinberg, "Goal setting and performance in sport and exercise settings: a synthesis and critique," *Medicine & Science in Sports & Exercise,* v. 26, April 1994, pp. 469–77.

James Annesi, "Goal-setting protocol in adherence to exercise by Italian adults," *Perception and Motor Skills,* v. 94, April 2002, pp. 453–58.

A. O. Booth, et al., "Dietary approaches for weight loss with increased fruit, vegetables and dairy," *Asia Pacific Journal of Clinical Nutrition,* Supplement, 2003, p. S10.

WEEK 1

MONDAY: Shawn Youngstedt, Daniel Kripke, and Jeffrey Elliott, "Is sleep disturbed by vigorous late-night exercise?" *Medicine & Science in Sports & Exercise,* v. 31, June 1999, pp. 864–69.

FRIDAY: Mihaela Tanasescu et al., "Exercise type and intensity in relation to coronary heart disease in men," *Journal of the American Medical Association,* v. 288, October 23, 2002, pp. 1994–2000.

WEEK 2

WEDNESDAY: "FDA Nutrition Labeling Manual: A Guide for Developing and Using Data Bases," 1998 Edition, U.S. Food and Drug Administration,

Center for Food Safety and Applied Nutrition, http://vm.cfsan.fda.gov/ ~dms/nutrguid.html.

THURSDAY: "Speed of Animals," *Natural History,* March 1974. The American Museum of Natural History and James G. Doherty, general curator, The Wildlife Conservation Society, www.infoplease.com/ipa/A0004737.html.

FRIDAY: Garry J Egger, Neeltje Vogels, and Klaas R Westerterp, "Estimating historical changes in physical activity levels," *Medical Journal of Australia,* 2001, v. 175, pp. 635–36.

David Bassett, et al., "Physical activity in an Old Order Amish community," *Medicine & Science in Sports & Exercise,* v. 36, January 2004, pp. 79–85.

SATURDAY: "A Position Statement on: Phytochemicals: Guardians of Our Health," General Conference Nutrition Council, Seventh Day Adventist Church, http://nadadventist.org/hm3/7020/gcnc/phyto/phyto.html.

WEEK 3

WEDNESDAY: N. C. Howarth, E. Saltzman, and Susan Roberts, "Dietary fiber and weight regulation," *Nutrition Review,* v. 59, May 2001, pp. 129–39.

Susan B. Roberts, Megan A. McCrory, and Edward Saltzman, "The influence of dietary composition on energy intake and body weight," *Journal of the American College of Nutrition,* v. 21, April 2002, pp. 141S-142S.

THURSDAY: "Death Valley's Incredible Weather," U.S. Geological Survey, National Parks Service, http://wrgis.wr.usgs.gov/docs/parks/deva/weather.html.

FRIDAY: Miriam Nelson, et al., "Effects of high-intensity strength training on multiple risk factors for osteoporotic fractures," *Journal of the American Medical Association,* v. 272, December 28, 1994, pp. 1909–14.

SATURDAY: Michael Jacobson and Jayne Hurley, *Restaurant Confidential* (Washington, D.C.: Center for Science in the Public Interest, 2001), pp. 211, 210, 226.

SUNDAY: "History of Swimming," Wikipedia, www.en.wikipedia.org/wiki/History_of_swimming.

WEEK 4

THURSDAY: "State-Specific Prevalence of Participation in Physical Activity," *Morbidity and Mortality Weekly Report,* Centers for Disease Control and Prevention, August 9, 1996, pp. 673–75, www.cdc.gov/epo/mmwr/preview/mmwrhtml/00043245.htm.

FRIDAY: James F. Clapp III and Eleanor Capeless, "The VO2 max of recreational athletes before and after pregnancy," *Medicine & Science in Sports & Exercise,* v. 23, October 1991, pp. 1128–33.

SUNDAY: "History of Women in Sports Timeline, Part 1—to 1899," St. Lawrence County Branch of the American Association of University Women, www.northnet.org/stlawrenceaauw/timeline.htm.

WEEK 5

WEDNESDAY: "Position of the American Dietetic Association: health implications of dietary fiber," *Journal of the American Dietetic Association,* v. 102, July 2002, pp. 993–1000.

THURSDAY: Metropolitan Police Recruit Physical Fitness Standards, Honolulu Police Department, www.honolulupd.org/hrd/fitness.htm.

Physical Fitness Requirements, Ohio Country Sheriff's Department, http://users.1st.net/ovdtf/ocsdfit.html.

FRIDAY: W. D. Schmidt, C. J. Biwer, et al., "Effects of long versus short bout exercise on fitness and weight loss in overweight females," *Journal of the American College of Nutrition,* v. 20, October 2001, pp. 494–501.

SUNDAY: Janice Todd, "The Strength Builders: A History of Barbells, Dumbbells, and Indian Clubs," *International Journal of the History of Sport,* v. 3, March 2003, pp. 65–90.

WEEK 6

WEDNESDAY: Lisa R. Young and Marion Nestle, "Expanding portion sizes in the U.S. marketplace: implications for nutrition counseling," *American Journal of Public Health,* v. 92, February 2002, pp. 246–49.

THURSDAY: Kirsten Weir, "Too cool: cold-water marathon swimmer Lynne Cox made the ultimate splash—in Antarctica," *Current Science,* August 29, 2003.

FRIDAY: M. R. Rhea, "The effects of competition and the presence of an audience on weight lifting performance," *Journal of Strength and Conditioning Research,* v. 17, May 2003, pp. 303–6.

SUNDAY: The Origins and Early History of Tennis, www.tennis.about.com/library/weekly/aa041101.htm.

WEEK 7

TUESDAY: F. Bellisle, R. McDevitt, et al., "Meal frequency and energy balance," *British Journal of Nutrition,* v. 77, Supplement 1, April 1997, pp. S57-S70.

WEDNESDAY: G. D. Foster, H. R. Wyatt, et al., "A randomized trial of a low-carbohydrate diet for obesity," *New England Journal of Medicine,* v. 348, May 2003, pp. 2082–90.

F. F. Samaha, N. Igbal, et al., "A low-carbohydrate as compared with a low-fat diet in severe obesity," *New England Journal of Medicine,* v. 348, May 2003, pp. 2074–81.

THURSDAY: "Economic Benefits of Physical Activity," World Health Organization, Noncommunicable Disease Prevention and Health Promotion, www.who.int/hpr/physactiv/economic.benefits.shtml.

FRIDAY: B. W. Wang, et al., "Postponed development of disability in elderly runners: a 13-year longitudinal study," *Archives of Internal Medicine,* v. 162, November 11, 2002, pp. 2285–94.

SUNDAY: Mel Siff, "A Short History of Strength and Conditioning," www.dolfzine.com/page515.htm.

WEEK 8

TUESDAY: R. J. Giorcelli and R. E. Hughes, "The effect of wearing a back belt on spine kinematics during asymmetric lifting of large and small boxes," *Spine,* v. 26, August 15, 2001, pp. 1794–98.

WEDNESDAY: Bonnie Liebman, "Ingredient Secrets," *Nutrition Action Health-letter,* Center for Science in the Public Interest, July/August 2001, p. 8.

THURSDAY: "The History of the Marathon," www.marathonguide.com/history/index.cfm.

FRIDAY: P. F. Kokkinos, "Exercise and hypertension," *Coronary Artery Disease,* v. 11, March 2000, pp. 99–102.

SATURDAY: Bonnie Liebman, "Ingredient Secrets," *Nutrition Action Health-letter,* Center for Science in the Public Interest, July/August 2001, p. 14.

SUNDAY: "The Free Dictionary.com: Bikini," www.encyclopedia.thefreedictionary.com/Bikini.

WEEK 9

TUESDAY: William D. McArdle, Frank I. Katch, and Victor L. Katch, "Top 12 Exercises Ranked by Relative Strenuousness," *Sports & Exercise Nutrition* (Lippincott, Wilkins & Williamson: Baltimore, 1999), p. 132.

"Aquatic Exercise Estimates METs and kcals for Men and Women," Aquatic Exercise Association, YMCA Water Fitness for Health, www.aeawave.com, North Venice, Florida.

THURSDAY: "Bicycling Magazine's Tour de France 2003, Just the Facts," www.tourdefrancenews.com/tourdefrance/facts/article/0,3493,4367,00.html.

FRIDAY: Eugenia Calle and Carmen Rodgriguez, "Overweight, obesity, and mortality from cancer in a prospectively studied cohort of U.S. adults," *New England Journal of Medicine,* v. 348, April 24, 2003, pp. 1625–38.

SUNDAY: "A Quick History of Bicycles," Pedaling History Bicycle Museum, www.pedalinghistory.com/PHhistory.html.

WEEK 10

THURSDAY: Ralph K. Requa, L. Nicole DeAvilla, and James G. Garrick, "Injuries in Recreational Adult Fitness Activities," *The American Journal of Sports Medicine,* v. 21, May–June 1993, pp. 461–67.

FRIDAY: "Clinical Guidelines on the identification, evaluation, and treatment of overweight and obesity in adults: the evidence report," NIH Publication No. 98–4083, 1998, National Institutes of Health, Bethesda, Maryland.

SUNDAY: Andrew Oon, "History of Swimming: Butterfly," Penang Amateur Swimming Association, www.penangswimming.com/main/sports/sub_sport_butterfly.html.

WEEK II

WEDNESDAY: "A Position Statement on: Phytochemicals: Guardians of Our Health," General Conference Nutrition Council, Seventh Day Adventist Church, http://nadadventist.org/hm3/7020/gcnc/phyto/phyto.html.

FRIDAY: Alisha L. Brosse, Erin S. Sheets, et al., "Exercise and the Treatment of Clinical Depression in Adults: Recent Findings and Future Directions," *Sports Medicine*, v. 32, 2002, pp. 741–60.

SUNDAY: Francesco Stefanon, "The Hawaii Ironman History," The Sport Web, www.geocities.com/hotsprings/3257/tristory.html.

WEEK 12

WEDNESDAY: Walter C. Willet and Meir J. Stampfer, "Rebuild the Food Pyramid," *Scientific American*, January 2003, pp. 64–71.

FRIDAY: Shawn Youngstedt, Patrick J. O'Connor, and Rod K. Dishman, "The effects of Acute Exercise on Sleep: A Quantitative Synthesis," *Sleep*, v. 20, March 1997, pp. 203–14.

Shawn Youngstedt, Michael L. Perlis, et al., "No association of sleep with total daily physical activity in normal sleepers," *Physiology & Behavior*, v. 78, March 2003, pp. 395–401.

SATURDAY: Bonnie Liebman and Margo Wootan, "Trans Fat," Nutrition Action Healthletter, June 1999, www.cspinet.org/nah/6_99/transfat3.html.

SUNDAY: Steven Vogel, "A short history of muscle-powered machines: what goes around comes around—and does useful work," *Natural History*, March 2002, www.findarticles.com/cf_dls/m1134/2_111/83553543/print.jhtml.

WEEK 13

THURSDAY: Simon Miller, "Down Under Up Top: Aussie Breaks 10-minute Mark," New York Sports Online, www.nysol.com/esbru.html.

FRIDAY: Frank Hu, et al., "Walking compared with vigorous physical activity and risk of type 2 diabetes in women: a prospective study," *Journal of the American Medical Association*, v. 343, October 20, 1999, pp. 1433–39.

WEEK 14

THURSDAY: "Calories burned during exercise," http://www.shapefit.com/calories.html.

FRIDAY: Dawnine Enette Larson-Meyer, "Effect of postpartum exercise on mothers and their offspring: a review of the literature," *Obesity Research*, v. 10, August 2002, pp. 841–53.

SUNDAY: Harvey Green, *Fit for America: Health, Fitness, Sport and American Society* (New York: Pantheon Books, 1986), p. 232.

WEEK 15

WEDNESDAY: David C. Nieman and Bente K. Pedersen, "Exercise and immune function: recent developments," *Sports Medicine*, v. 27, February 1999, pp. 73–80.

FRIDAY: Miriam Nelson and Sarah Wernick, *Strong Women Stay Young* (New York: Bantam Books, 2000), p. 12.

SATURDAY: Bonnie Liebman and Jayne Hurley, "The Food Court: Guilty or Innocent?" *Nutrition Action Healthletter*, Center for Science in the Public Interest, April 2001, pp. 1–9.

SUNDAY: Edward Norman Gardiner, *Athletics of the Ancient World* (Oxford, England: Oxford University Press, 1930), p. 44.

WEEK 16

FRIDAY: Miriam E. Nelson with Sarah Wernick, *Strong Women, Strong Bones* (New York: Perigee, 1999), p. 150.

SUNDAY: David E. Martin and Roger W. H. Gynn, *The Olympic Marathon: The*

History and Drama of Sport's Most Challenging Event (Champaign: Human Kinetics, 2000), pp. 5–6 and 57–58.

WEEK 17

WEDNESDAY: Mitch Lipka, "Many Food Labels Are Incorrect: Errors in 'Nutritional Facts' Panels May Be Hazardous To Health of Consumers," *South Florida Sun–Sentinel,* September 2, 2001, p. 1.A.

FRIDAY: "Report on Weight-Loss Advertising: An Analysis of Current Trends," Federal Trade Commission, September 2002, www.ftc.gov/opa/2002/09/weightlossrpt.htm.

SATURDAY: "Cheesecake's carrot cake latest target of CSPI ire," *Nation's Restaurant News,* July 2, 2001, www.findarticles.com/cf_dls/m3190/27_35/76447603/p1/article.jhtml.

SUNDAY: "Interesting Olympic Facts," www.history1900s.about.com/library/misc/blolympicfacts.htm.

WEEK 18

FRIDAY: J. P. Wallace, "Twelve month adherence of adults who joined a fitness program with a spouse vs. without a spouse," *Journal of Sports Medicine and Physical Fitness,* v. 35, September 1995, pp. 206–13.

SUNDAY: "Fact Monster: Golf" www.factmonster.com/ipka/A0768372.html.

WEEK 19

WEDNESDAY: Nelson, *Strong Women, Strong Bones,* p. 25.

SUNDAY: "History of Pole Vaulting," www.health.howstuffworks.com/pole-vault.htm.

WEEK 20

THURSDAY: David Bassett, et al., "Physical activity in an Old Order Amish community," *Medicine & Science in Sports & Exercise,* v. 36, January 2004, pp. 79–85.

FRIDAY: Frank Hu, et al., "Physical activity and television watching in relation to risk for type 2 diabetes mellitus in men," *Archives of Internal Medicine*, v. 161, June 25, 2001, pp. 1542–48.

SUNDAY: "History of Soccer," Tetra Brazil Soccer Academy, www.tetrabrazil.com/history_of_soccer.htm.

WEEK 21

THURSDAY: "Amazing Feats of Strength," Guinness Book of World Records, www.guinnessworldrecords.com/index.asp?id=56773.

FRIDAY: James F. Clapp III, *Exercising Through Your Pregnancy* (Champaign: Human Kinetics, 1998), pp. 93–95.

SUNDAY: "History of Swimming," Wikipedia, www.en.wikipedia.org/wiki/History_of_swimming.

WEEK 22

TUESDAY: W. D. Bandy, J. M. Irion, and M. Briggler, "The effect of static stretch and dynamic range of motion training on the flexibility of the hamstring muscles," *The Journal of Orthopaedic and Sports Physical Therapy*, v. 27, April 1998, pp. 295–300.

THURSDAY: "Swimming Speeds of Some Common Fish," National Maritime Research Institute, www.nmri.go.jp/eng/khirata/fish/general/speed/speede.htm.

FRIDAY: L. Marceau, et al., "Does bicycling contribute to the risk of erectile dysfunction? Results from the Massachusetts Male Aging Study," *International Journal of Impotence Research*, v. 13, October 2001, pp. 298–302.

SUNDAY: "History of Yoga — A Complete Overview of the History of Yoga," www.abc-of-yoga.com/beginnersguide/yogahistory.asp.

WEEK 23

THURSDAY: "RAAM Riders Lose More Fat," Cycling Calorie News, www.pwp.value.net/%7Efitness/cycnews#1.

FRIDAY: Edward McAuley, et al., "Cardiovascular fitness and neurocognitive function in older adults: a brief review," *Brain Behavior Immunology*, v. 18, May 2004, pp. 214–20.

SUNDAY: "History of the Sport of Gymnastics," www.shrike.depaul.edu/ ~vbard/histpg.html.

WEEK 24

THURSDAY: "Prevalence of Physical Activity, Including Lifestyle Activities Among Adults: United States, 2000–2001," *Morbidity and Mortality Weekly Report,* August 15, 2003, pp. 764–69.

FRIDAY: S. L. Wong, "Cardiorespiratory Fitness Is Associated with Lower Abdominal Fat Independent of Body Mass Index," *Medicine & Science in Sports & Exercise,* v. 36, February 2004, pp. 286–91.

SUNDAY: Harvey Green, *Fit for America: Health, Fitness, Sport and American Society* (New York: Pantheon Books, 1986), pp. 99 and 184.